Zandra

My Daughter, Diabetes, and Lessons in Love

JANET HATCH

Zandra

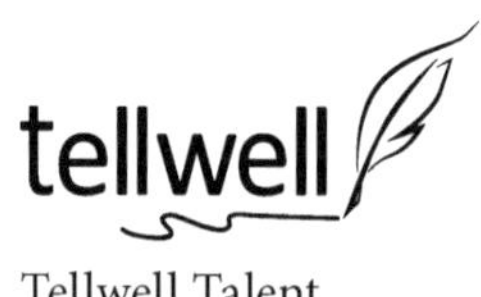

Tellwell Talent
www.tellwell.ca

ISBN
978-0-2288-3702-2 (Paperback)
978-0-2288-3703-9 (eBook)

To my family, Gord, Zandra, Olivia, Joseph and Liam: Thank you for journeying in this life with me. You have given me the opportunity to grow and expand my awareness in infinite ways. Through your presence and love, I have had the opportunity to see the world through your unique and beautiful eyes and by doing so, heal old wounds and find self-love.

CHAPTER 1

The Diagnosis

"What's the reason for your visit?" The admitting nurse at our tiny local hospital was staring at me impatiently while my eleven-year-old daughter, Zandra, shuffled nervously at my side.

"She's showing signs of type 1 diabetes," I explained, the words sounding unbelievable as I said them out loud.

"Well, we'll see," the nurse huffed in frustration. "We don't appreciate people looking up "Doctor Google" before they get here; that's the job of the actual doctor." She tapped heavily on her keyboard while processing the paperwork. "We don't have time for everyone who thinks something is wrong because they looked it up on the internet."

Normally I would be upset at being administered a tongue-lashing, but this time I was too worried about Zandra. I wanted my theory to be wrong, and I'd take a curt retort any day over being right this time.

After spending what felt like several hours in the waiting room, the doctor finally appeared. He commented on Zandra's appearance. He noted the dark circles under her eyes, her underweight frame and pallid colour. He immediately ordered a blood requisition, and within a half hour he returned to give us her diagnosis. "Her blood sugars are extremely elevated, and she has ketones in her urine," he explained. "I'm sorry to have to tell you this, but she has type 1 diabetes."

The doctor's words sent a vibration throughout my body that threatened to buckle me at my knees. I felt an instant, surreal shock which only confirmed what my intuition had already told me. As I began to absorb the information, I asked if there was any way she could get a single shot of insulin to balance her body, returning it to normal. He explained that there was no going back, that her blood sugars wouldn't return to normal without lifelong insulin therapy. He explained that although she was sick, he'd seen kids worse off. He commended me on noticing the signs and bringing her in. He asked Zandra if she had any questions about her diagnosis, but I'm sure he realized that she likely didn't know what her diagnosis even meant—she was only eleven years old. I didn't tell him about the nurse. A part of me wanted to lash out and direct my pain on the easiest target, but I knew that the momentary satisfaction of doing so wouldn't change Zandra's diagnosis. We were told that the children's hospital in Edmonton was full and that we would have to spend the night in the Camrose hospital and be transferred the next day. The hospital staff quickly set us up in a private room, where I told Zandra my story of growing up with a diabetic dog and how I helped to care for her. I also shared with her about having a diabetic boyfriend in high school and how I saw firsthand how such a diagnosis could coexist within a happy, full life. Throughout my experiences I had learned a lot about diabetes and was able to provide her with at least a rudimentary explanation of the disease.

I started by explaining the difference between type 1 and type 2 diabetes. I didn't want her to feel that she had done anything to cause her illness. I explained that type 1 diabetes (which was previously known as juvenile diabetes) was an autoimmune disease whereby little or no insulin is produced by the pancreas. I told her that insulin is an important hormone needed for the body to process blood sugar and that she would now always require a needle in order for her body to get that same hormone. I told her that many people have type 2 diabetes; however, this is most often developed in adults, and although they require insulin, their body still produces some itself. Type 2 diabetes isn't an autoimmune disease, and for many people it can be controlled by diet and exercise.

Before we left the emergency room to move to our new room on a different unit, the admitting nurse came to me. She had heard the doctor's diagnosis and apologized for her comments. I imagine she was wishing she could take them back. Her apology comforted me. I knew it took courage on her part and I could see the empathy on her face. I needed a friendly face—hers would have to do.

Becoming a mother for me meant learning what it was to love someone so much that you would lay your life on the line without a second's thought. The feeling that a part of my heart and soul lay outside of myself made me vulnerable like nothing else. I feel everything that happens to my child, whether good or bad, in my own soul. Simply put: when my child is hurt, I hurt. Everything before the diagnosis felt simpler. Nothing we had ever dealt with had had the same impact as diabetes. I questioned my role and my qualifications to be the parent I needed to be, and the parent Zandra deserved to have.

I wondered if something I had done—or not done—had contributed to her diagnosis. Thoughts swirled in my mind, whether I had taken enough prenatal vitamins when I was pregnant with her or given her enough vitamins as a baby. I tormented myself endlessly those first days, trying to figure out where I went wrong so I could try to make it right.

I worried for my other children as well—Olivia, who was two years younger than Zandra, and Joseph, who was born a couple of years after that. Liam came a while later; he was over ten years younger than Zandra. I had experienced high blood pressure during my pregnancies with Olivia and Joseph, which created their own complications; however, each baby was different from the others. Olivia—Liv, as we call her—had been a textbook baby, other than some colic. She followed the growth charts and milestones perfectly, and apart from some flus and ear infections, she rarely became sick. Joseph, however, was different. Soon after his birth, he was taken to intensive care where he nearly died. All of his little systems seemed to be failing for no apparent reason. His condition worsened until his fifth day of life when, by some miracle, he ended up pulling through and was able to come home on Christmas Eve. In Joseph's early years, he struggled with persistent ear infections, which thankfully resolved as he got older. With Liam, my fourth child, my pregnancy was as healthy as he was. He was my biggest baby at 9 pounds 3 ounces, and he achieved his own milestones according to his own timeline. With more experience, I became increasingly comfortable with my babies moving along the charts in their own timing, without feeling that they were somehow ahead or behind the anticipated curve.

Much of my life as a parent prior to diabetes had consisted of balancing the routines and schedules of everyone in our household: meals, school and work, naps and appointments. Days and weeks moved along quickly under the momentum of daily lives. My life could be set into autopilot when I needed to rest and turned on a dime with little disruption to anyone else. Like a pro athlete, I knew how to plan, prepare and navigate whatever came my way—until diabetes.

Nothing had prepared me for my new role. There wasn't a name that defined the change in my life. Caregiver? I've always cared for my children. Nurse? I wasn't qualified, yet I felt different from the parent I was before the diagnosis. I was filling a role that needed all my abilities and could have dire consequences if I didn't perform them well. I had heard from parents who'd had children pass away that there wasn't a name to define their loss, no name with substance enough to explain that they once gave a piece of their soul to another who was no longer there. As with the loss of a child, I struggled with language to identify the raw nerve that was outside of myself, sending signals to me night and day that my daughter's life was in a delicate balance.

When soccer season came to an end just before the summer Zandra was diagnosed, Zandra looked tired and skinny. I assumed the reason was that she had been quite active for several months and needed a rest. Summer break was just what we needed. I noticed that she had large dark circles around her eyes, the same ones that indicated she needed to check her diet. We needed to make sure that we went back to the restricted diet that she had been following since she was two years old, when she developed a soy, wheat and milk sensitivity. As she got older, it seemed that we were pulling away from it and the thought crossed my mind that her physical appearance may have been the reminder we needed to be strict with her diet. I needed to make an appointment to check her vitamin D levels, as they had been checked a year prior and were found to be seriously low, but life got busy and my to-do's got tabled for another month.

The beginning of the summer before Zandra's diagnosis was beautiful. We found our groove and decided to take a trip to Banff

National Park, nestled in the Rocky Mountains, one of our family's favourite destinations. Liam was just learning to walk and was able to enjoy almost all the activities that summer would provide. Zandra invited her friend Maiya to join us. We planned to go river rafting, horseback riding and hiking through the mountain trails. We even brought our old dog, Murphy. Murphy was a husky crossed with a lot of things. He loved his family and never wanted to miss a road trip. One of the many highlights of our trip was frequenting one of the quintessential downtown sweet shops that greeted its patrons with a small-town feeling and hand-crafted chocolates. This was something we always made a stop for when visiting. The kids loved the names of the chocolates: "moose droppings"—chocolate-covered almonds—and "bear paws," which featured cashews as the claws. This vacation was by all accounts one of our family favourites.

That summer would end up being our last with our beloved Murphy. He was just shy of his fourteenth birthday and his kidneys had been failing for some time. Although we had been taking care of him with the help and guidance of our vet, we knew the time was close to saying goodbye. We had watched him slow down with arthritis for the last year, and he would often set out on a walk with the enthusiasm of a pup, only to get part way and have his hind end give out on him, his arthritis betraying his puppy-like sense of adventure. During the last month, we were encouraged to walk with him in the baby stroller to keep him happy and emotionally satisfied. I would place our sixty-pound dog in the baby stroller, attach Liam to the baby carrier on my chest and set out for daily walks. We were watching Murphy closely to know when he wasn't coping well. The day came sooner than we wanted it to. It was the opening day of the Big Valley Jamboree in our hometown of Camrose, which was an annual music festival that brings celebrity country singers and their fans together for a three-day festival. The kick-off parade was about to start, and we were all getting ready to head downtown for the festivities. Before we left, we let Murphy outside to have a chance to relieve himself before we went out. Murphy couldn't climb out onto the stairs of the deck. He appeared to be confused when we called for him, and he didn't seem to understand how to do such a routine task. That was the day we called the vet and took Murphy for his last car ride.

My husband, Gord, took the kids to the parade while I said my final farewell in private, and when the kids arrived home, I left with the girls and Murphy.

Dr. Copland had been Murphy's vet for several years. She genuinely cared for him and her affection was clear when she lay down on the carpet of the special room created to say goodbye to beloved pets and said her own farewell to Murphy. Her compassion moved me to tears. We were safe to let him go with her. She left Murphy to spend some last moments with us and indicated that she would come when we were ready to let him pass. We shared tears and stories as we hugged and kissed our old boy, who was clearly ready to leave his tired body. This was the first loss for the girls and the grief was like losing a child for me. Murphy had been with me for over thirteen years, since the day of my dad's funeral, and was by my side through two marriages and four children. We were a team and I couldn't fathom my life without him. Murphy knew me better than any human ever had. He knew my secrets and had loved me unconditionally his entire life.

When the girls and I came home without Murphy, we felt raw. Our house wasn't the same. Our hearts felt tremendous grief at such a loss. I could hear weeping from Zandra's, Liv's and Joseph's rooms throughout the night. Nothing I could say or do could console them. I just let them sit with their loss as they tried to reconcile their feelings. They struggled to process their grief and discover their new normal without Murphy. They would experience loss again, in time, and as hard as it was, it was part of the human experience. I knew that eventually we would be able to share in the beautiful memories we made with him. As a mom, watching my children grieve was agony. Looking back, I see now that the loss we shared was beautiful. I was grateful to Murphy for teaching me that I wasn't alone—none of us were. We had each other and I felt connected through our grief.

I worried about the hurt that each of the children had to cope with since my divorce with Kelley, their dad. We had been separated for over five years, when Joseph was just one year old, and I was keenly aware that my ability to maintain an amicable relationship with their dad would benefit them in immeasurable ways. Knowing that my decision would impact them so significantly added to my guilt that was already a greater burden than I could manage. It was important to me that the children maintain a relationship with Kelley, even though we now lived an hour away and I was remarried to Gord, who had instantly become a father to three.

Several days after losing Murphy, Zandra went to visit her friend Kendra for a sleepover. Both girls played for the same team and were equally competitive. I was happy for her to have the opportunity to get away, as her friend's mom, a friend of mine, was compassionate and fun-loving, and she knew about and understood our recent loss. I felt she would be exactly what Zandra needed as she moved on without Murphy. Zandra was excited to go. She had never had a sleepover with this friend before and was looking forward to it. The plan was that I would pick her up the next day and we would go straight to drop her, Olivia and Joseph off to see their dad for his upcoming week. Since the divorce, Kelley and I shared summers, rotating with the kids one week at a time. When I picked her up, she told me she was parched and asked for a snack as well. I asked her whether she had eaten breakfast and she indicated that she had but was still hungry. I was already on the way out of town with the other three kids packed and ready, so I didn't want to stop at home for food. I decided to head over to a gas station and pick her up something quick there. Zandra picked out and quickly inhaled a can of pop and a sandwich. She downed the drink in a couple of gulps and asked to refill it with water, but we were already on the highway. She complained a lot on the hour-long trip that she was thirsty. When we arrived at what's known as "Egg Park," the park in Vegreville with the world's largest Ukrainian pysanka (a decorated Easter egg), she ran into the public restroom, refilling her pop can several times and guzzling the water down like I had never seen her do before.

Something in me was very uneasy. This didn't feel right. Thoughts started coming to my mind, but I didn't want to give attention to them. I didn't want to drop her off; everything in me was telling me to keep her close, but nothing with enough certainty to say the words out loud. When I met Kelley at the park, I told him about Zandra. I asked that he keep a good eye on her, even though I knew he didn't pay the same attention to things that I did.

I said goodbye to the kids knowing I would see them in a week, hoping that all would be well during that time. I left the park watching the kids swinging with their dad on the monkey bars from the rear-view mirror of my navy-blue minivan. I had an hour to drive home with Liam, who was unusually quiet for the entire way back. The hour return trip provided the quiet I needed to listen to what my mind was trying to say. The thoughts seemed to be pulling together and connecting the way they hadn't when I was at the park. I was deeply regretting leaving Zandra behind. The symptoms began to unfold as I thought about the random yet strange physical ailments Zandra experienced over the last several months. I recalled just weeks earlier that she came to me with soiled sheets one morning before school, clearly upset what had happened. I then turned my mind to the vision loss she had been complaining about, which at the time I had attributed to late-night reading in bed. When added to the new list of ailments, a clearer picture began to form—all were pointing in one direction and setting off alarms in my mind. I didn't want this to be the message I was getting, but it all led me to one conclusion: Zandra had diabetes.

I could feel myself gasping for breath, making each one a challenge as I drove home. When I got there I immediately called Kelley, telling him what I understood in my gut to be true, but keeping a logical head for the sake of appearances. Kelley assured me that she was fine and no longer as thirsty. I desperately accepted his observations. He said he would keep an eye on her and let me know in a couple of days how things were going, or sooner if something was wrong. By the time I got home, Gord had arrived from work. I told him about my fears, about the thirst and her symptoms, and how anxious I was. He reassured me that I was likely making more of things than I needed to. He encouraged me to give Kelley the benefit of the doubt and asked me how I would feel should the shoe be on the other foot. Gord always grounded me in times when I felt overwhelmed, and even though I still felt anxious about Zandra, I recognized that I needed to approach this and future interactions in a more tempered manner. Those next days were agony for me. I knew that I had to look reasonable for the kids and Kelley. Although we were keeping peace, I knew that if I appeared illogical or overstepping, he would act in kind and that was a battle I didn't want to start. I had worked too hard to get where we were and keeping Zandra where I could watch her would certainly create a wave that would overturn that ship.

I waited a couple of days and didn't hear anything from Kelley. I decided to call after contemplating it all morning. I didn't get an answer on the first try. The panic continued to elevate, so I called back two more times until he answered. He said they were at a birthday party and that Zandra was just fine. He explained that she was still thirsty, but he didn't feel as though it was serious. I wanted to talk to her directly, but Kelley said she was with Olivia and Joseph and eating birthday cake at that moment and wasn't able to talk to me. Something in me reacted. I knew something was wrong. I had been married to him long enough to know when he was keeping something from me. I told him that I wanted her to come home so I could see her for myself. He felt threatened and said that he wouldn't bring her. I didn't want to be irrational. I had no proof something was wrong, just what I was feeling in my heart. I felt scared and stuck. I was angry that I had to be diplomatic even when it came to our daughter's health. I realized that I needed to step up and try to see it from his perspective. In the end I just needed to know if Zandra was okay. We agreed that he would take her to the hospital to be checked and follow up with me. I paced the floor, waiting for an update that would take hours. After a while, I impatiently called back. Kelley informed me that he hadn't taken her to the hospital, but he had taken her to the drug store where the pharmacist tested her blood sugars with a blood glucose tester. He said that the tester came back unreadable, so they figured it malfunctioned and decided to leave it at that. Apparently, nobody had thought to retest her.

I was in a full panic. The knot in my stomach threatened to burst open. I told Kelley that I was extremely concerned and wanted to pick her up. "You can take her to the clinic on your week with the kids," he snarked. Risking all the peace we'd worked for, I threatened to call the police. I knew that even if I was reprimanded the police would likely pursue her health condition, and I would know for sure whether what I feared was true or not, and if it was that she would get the help she needed immediately. This threat came out so quickly and without warning that all I could do was listen to the words coming from my own mouth. I surprised myself. Kelley didn't want me *or* the police showing up, so he said he would bring her to me.

An hour later, I met Kelley just outside of town. Zandra looked terrible. She was visibly worse than she had been when I dropped her off. I went immediately to the Camrose hospital to have her looked at by a doctor and was in no mood to deal with the snarky admitting nurse we encountered there. After spending what felt like several hours in the waiting room, and after dealing with a heated call with Zandra's father, the doctor finally appeared. While we were waiting, Kelley called and suggested I hold off getting a diagnosis to take out a life insurance plan for her first. He said his reasoning was because his friend's child had been diagnosed with diabetes, and as he was entering adulthood he was finding it hard to afford insurance with his pre-existing condition. In his eyes, this advice was helpful and pragmatic, but to me it demonstrated clearly where his priorities lay, and why I could not trust his judgment.

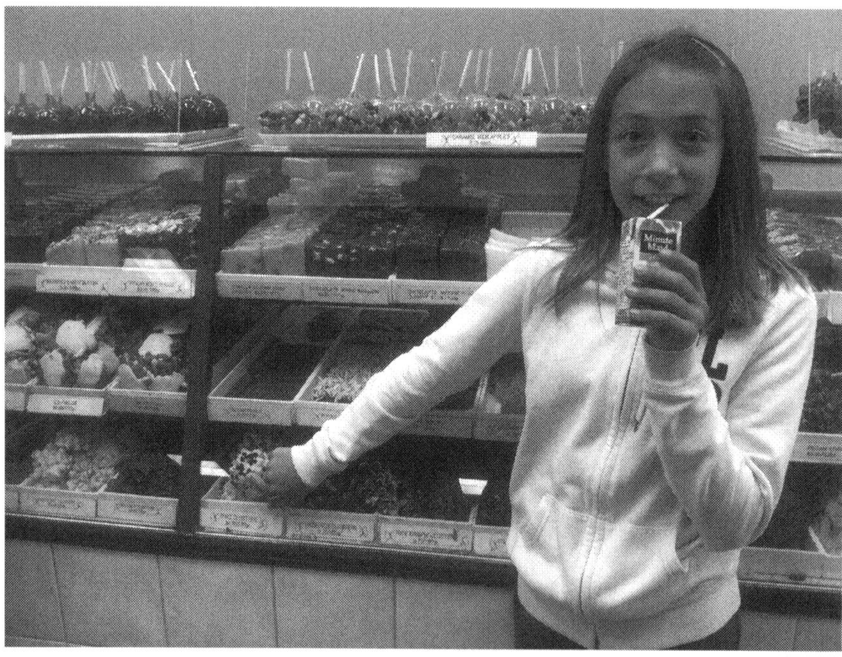

Zandra at the sweet-shop just weeks before diagnosis

CHAPTER 2

Alexandra

ALEXANDRA FAITH ARRIVED ON JANUARY 12, 2000. She was born with thick black hair and dark olive skin, and weighed 7 pounds 4 ounces. Motherhood proved exhausting after experiencing thirty-eight hours of hard labour. I felt depleted, scared and excited all at the same time. I was in awe just holding her in my arms after a long pregnancy and delivery.

I chose the name Alexandra after watching the movie *Alex: The Life of a Child* when I was ten years old. The movie was a true story of a spunky little girl born with cystic fibrosis. The little girl, who died at only eight years old, showed the world and her family how to live and love in her short life. As I sat in front of our old cabinet TV, I was captivated that a child of a similar age could endure so much and have her life taken away so young. It was powerful. The story seemed to resonate deeply within me. Alex had a disease for which there was no cure, and in the end nobody could save her. Her name became imprinted on my heart with curiosity and purpose. I knew God loved children and would call them home, yet it always felt strange to me. I wondered why he chose some and not others? I wondered if I would be chosen, and if so, for what reason? From then on, I always named my dolls Alex, and became "Alexandra" when I was role-playing. I chose her middle name, Faith, not only as it was a namesake from my mom's youngest sister, Virginia Faith, but also because I had faith that God created me for a powerful purpose unknown to me, faith I felt strongly.

Alexandra was born at 9:07 p.m. By the time she had been checked over by the nurses and returned to me, it was after eleven. I was exhausted and so was Kelley. The exhaustion caught up with Kelley and his asthma began to act up. He was struggling for some time while I was in labour, so after a while he went downstairs to the emergency unit for some medication to help, then headed home for a proper sleep so he would be healthy and refreshed for his new family the next day. From the first night, Alexandra was fussy and wouldn't settle. It seemed as if she was born angry, and deep down I felt she had been.

I had experienced a lot of exhaustion and frustration during my pregnancy with her, for which I felt immense guilt. On top of that, I didn't feel comfortable with babies. The agitation I was feeling carried over to her. I felt exhausted and my ability to cope was diminishing with each passing hour. I rang for the nurses to come and take her from me. A nurse swiftly responded to my bedside call and I asked if she could take my baby so I could sleep and be spelled off. I could feel her reply before she spoke the words. She explained that they don't have nurseries in hospitals anymore and that I needed to get used to being a mother and looking after the baby myself. My defences were down and all I felt was the shame of being a young mother who couldn't cope on the first day. At twenty-three, I looked young and was being treated as such. I felt shame for having asked and humiliated by her response. I managed to stand up and rock Alexandra, finding it the only way she would settle. With my legs still partially numb from the epidural I had been given hours before, I spent most of the night standing and rocking so the fussing wouldn't wake my roommate and her sleeping baby.

In the early morning I managed some rest just before the doctor came in for a routine check of the baby. For the first time, I began unwrapping her swaddled blanket to peek at her tiny fingers and toes. I counted all of them to be sure that all were there. When I got to her left foot, I didn't see any toes, I just saw a peg where her foot should be. I searched frantically for her other foot, wondering why nobody had told me that she was deformed. I grew frantic. As the doctor was organizing his papers, he saw my distress. He approached me and told me that her foot was twisted and what looked like a peg for a leg was, in fact, her heel. He assured me that she had all her toes on each foot. Her tiny foot was so twisted that her heel pointed downward, and her foot was twisted completely around so that the top of her toes touched her shin. The doctor warned me that her foot would need to be looked at by a specialist so that she could walk properly. I felt enormous relief. This I could handle. I too was born with a twisted left foot and, although I never saw it at birth, I never felt it was significant. I suffered with pain, swelling and a bone that protruded like a bunion for as long as I could remember. I had pain from not treating it properly, something I would never let happen to my own daughter. Growing up I was often told "you'll soldier on," so my pain was dismissed. I felt huge relief. After all that could have gone wrong, a twisted foot wasn't the worst diagnosis.

After the doctor left, I resolved to face the day with a fresh shower. I put on a hospital robe and wheeled Alexandra to the nurses' desk to have them watch her so I could use the restroom. There was a different nurse there than the one from the night shift, but she repeated the mantra of the last one. I was told that there wouldn't be a nurse to watch her when I left the hospital, so I had to learn how to shower with a baby. I was told I couldn't leave her alone in the room and to take her in the bathroom with me. I wanted to sink into the floor. I felt so ashamed all over again. I was already feeling like the worst mother on the unit and now I had confirmed it. I wheeled my baby back to my room and squeezed the infant bed into the bathroom to set about having a record-fast shower—something that would become the normal routine for many years. I managed a functional shower and proved to myself and the nurses that I was capable of managing the most menial of tasks. This was all foreign to me. Everything was painful, although in the end the shower perked me up and allowed me to face my new life as a mother. I resolved to start fresh, leaving behind my shame and insecurities to drain out with the old bathwater.

The next nurse who arrived was concerned about feeding the baby. She was much kinder than the others I'd had so far. She guided me to properly latch the baby to nurse her. It took more practice than I thought, but I got the hang of it and so did Alexandra. After a while on my breast, the nurse picked up Alexandra to show me how to properly burp her. While she was holding her, she was troubled by the way Alexandra was breathing. She manoeuvred her to see if burping her would clear up the airways, but it didn't. She quickly called the doctor back to have a look at her. While the doctor was examining her, the nurse asked me how long she had been breathing like that. Strike three for me. I didn't even notice that her breathing was off. I explained that I had been with her the entire morning and it had sounded what I thought was normal. I told them about the shower, thinking that the moist air was helpful—otherwise why would I have been instructed to take her in with me? I was immediately chastised by the consulting doctor for taking a newborn into a humid environment. I explained that I was told to bring her in and wasn't given a choice, yet he gave me a disapproving look. Alexandra had to be taken away for several hours for observation and later put on antibiotics to clear up what may have been the start of pneumonia in her lungs. I couldn't possibly feel any more like a failure. I was told that she needed to stay another night to be sure that it wouldn't get any worse. Motherhood was proving to be a journey that I was not equipped for.

By afternoon, baby Alexandra was well enough to greet some visitors. Her great-grandparents, aunts, uncles and only cousin, Erick, all came to meet our newest family member. Some of my coworkers and friends also came to meet her. With the name Alexandra, a lot of people shorten the name to Alex. Some of the new visitors already had, but I wanted to be a bit different. We thought of shortening it to Ally or Lexi, but those didn't feel right. Another shortened name suggested in the baby book I brought with me was Zandra. I loved it immediately. This little dark-haired and olive-skinned baby seemed exotic to me and needed a more exotic name. The name felt perfect. She still had the name I always cherished yet a personal alias that suited her own unique being.

By the morning of her third day, Zandra had been given the all-clear to leave the hospital. After filling out the paperwork and going through car-seat checks, Kelley and I were on our way home with our new baby. The ride home felt long. Zandra was fussy for most of it, and with over an hour to drive, my nerves were frayed by the time we arrived. Coming home was exciting, however, as Zandra was able to meet the rest of our family: our dogs, Bear and Murphy. The dogs were excited to see me after several days being away and were quite interested in this new little human I had brought home. They were instinctively cautious with her, and although I found Bear sleeping in her bassinette on occasion, he never climbed in with her. The dogs were in for a life change, just like we were.

The days and weeks following Zandra's arrival were difficult. I was struck with a headache like nothing else I've ever experienced. I couldn't believe how much a head could hurt. It was a struggle to perform my own daily functions, much less look after a baby and entertain visitors excited to see her. What I didn't know at the time was that I was experiencing a side effect from the epidural I had received at the final hour of Zandra's delivery. Although it was a great relief at the time, I was later told some people experience excruciating headaches afterward and that there was an injection available to counteract the side effects. However, I was fed up with doctors and didn't have the energy or motivation to get help. When the nurse came to the house for a wellness check, I put on a smile and let her know that everything was just fine. I would just have to soldier on.

Parenting was exhausting, but the sweet bundle that lay before me more than made up for it. My new role as a mother filled me with a sense of meaning that I could not describe. I felt pride that I had created such a beautiful human being. As much as I cherished my baby, it was also a challenge like none other I had faced. I had very little sleep and a fussy baby whenever her eyes were open. Nothing seemed to settle her. My mom had only ever visited a handful of times, but on one occasion her visit was a godsend. Zandra was only a couple of months old and I was exhausted. If I could name a skill of Mom's, it was to love babies. She seemed to have endless energy to waltz them across the living room until they settled. What she lacked in skills for taking care of older children, she more than made up for with caring for babies. Zandra was more than colicky; something wasn't right, and Mom identified it straight away. I had been breastfeeding Zandra and was careful to watch my diet, but Mom insisted that she couldn't handle the breast milk. It seemed unnatural to me, but upon her insistence I went to the store and bought a container of a soy-based formula. The results were amazing. I had supplemented her with bottles before, but as I had a lot of milk I knew hunger wasn't the problem. In that first week on the soy formula, the sleep that I got was more than in the first months combined. I decided that it was best for her as well as me if I fed her formula exclusively.

The decision to quit nursing was a difficult one. Overwhelming emotions of being an inadequate mom seeped into my thoughts and etched a trail of doubts. I worked hard to accept this decision to bottle feed, despite the overwhelming benefits of breastfeeding. At her next wellness check with her doctor, the paediatrician asked the routine question: "Are you breastfeeding or bottle feeding?" I explained about the switch to bottle and why I did it, and she quipped, "Don't tell me that. Breastfeeding is best." I felt my heart sink and my face blush with shame. My eyes burned and threatened to hail tears in the clinic office. I wanted someone to hug me and tell me that even the fact that I was trying was good for her. I knew in my heart that I loved and cared for my baby, yet I felt entirely unsupported. I knew I couldn't go back to this doctor. I needed to find someone who respected me and supported me. I called my younger sister Laura and told her about what had happened. She suggested I make an appointment with our childhood doctor, Dr. Tedishini. She said he was still practising and was also a teaching doctor at the university. I knew Laura was right. I wanted to take her advice, but I felt defeated. I didn't want to go to such a revered doctor only for him to find out that I was making mistakes. I didn't have the confidence to hear any more criticism, especially from someone I once knew. Instead, I told Laura that I would see a local physician, as the hour's drive to Edmonton was a lot for me.

Zandra, by all descriptions from the baby books I had read, was a strong-willed child. Growing up, my mom always said God would punish me with a child just like me, and it appeared he had. Zandra would challenge me on all occasions, from grocery shopping to bath time and everything in between. The unique challenge was also a thrill. The upside of having this strong-willed child was seeing myself. If I was anything as tenacious and bright as she was, I had potential. I wondered if my mom saw me through the same lens. This remarkable child was perfect in all her challenges and, although exhausting, had a sense of humour to match. One Christmas when she was almost two, she was upset with me and called me "a bad banana with a greasy black peel," as she had remembered it from *The Grinch* soundtrack. It was all I could do to keep a straight face. It was the funniest, not to mention most creative, thing that I had ever been called. It was the worst insult her innocent mind could conjure up.

On another occasion, when Zandra was in preschool, she was waiting for the bus and rebelling from the hurrying it took to get her ready. She turned around and told me that I had white hair and yellow teeth—something she had picked up on that adults don't want to have. Again, I wanted to laugh, but instead told her that speaking harsh words hurt my feelings and that she should think before she reacted in anger. She took another moment and gathered herself, only to come back with, "You have silver hair and golden teeth." I was so impressed with her wit and creativity I had nothing to reply with, other than a smile that assured her I understood her frustrations.

As Zandra grew, it seemed that she was sick more often than the other children in our circle. I noticed she was more susceptible to viruses, and when she was sick it seemed to always grow into a fever and ear infection. When I was pregnant with Olivia, things seemed to go downhill. Zandra was often complaining of stomach aches and was either constipated or cramped with diarrhea. She began regularly throwing up her food. She would develop dark circles under her eyes and a distended belly. I was avoiding all milk products, but nothing seemed to help. I had her into the local doctor for every test, but other than obvious gas in her belly, every test came back negative. The frequency of her vomiting was almost daily and seemed uncontrollable. On one occasion the vomiting got so bad she needed to be admitted into the hospital for dehydration. It was like she had a flu that wouldn't pass. I had no idea what was happening, nor did her doctor.

One day Zandra became so sick that she threw up all over her bookshelves, covering her books with vomit. She cherished her books, and this was devastating to her. She told me she wanted to die and let God take her to Heaven where there was no pain. Hearing this from a three-year-old was gut wrenching, not to mention from my own child. Indeed, I knew God brought children home. I started crying with her. I cleaned her up, leaving the shelves and her books still covered, and drove her straight to the clinic. I walked in and started crying. She had been sick every day for the best part of a year and nobody seemed to believe me or offer any suggestions. I found the courage to advocate and told the doctor that I wasn't leaving until I had a course of action, because I couldn't help a child who wanted to die. Her doctor admitted her into the hospital.

The difference between this visit and the last was that they were fasting her. They wanted to see if she was ingesting something that was making her sick. They knew she didn't have milk products, but a curious nurse insisted that this was the best course. She told me she understood my position, as she had gone through something similar with her son, and for him the culprit was eggs. After a couple of days on only an intravenous IV, Zandra wasn't vomiting. This was telling. When I returned to the local doctor, he insisted that, as her allergy tests had come back normal, there was nothing wrong with her. According to him, I had to let her grow out of it. He said he didn't believe in intolerances that couldn't be proven in blood tests. I hurriedly put on our coats, fighting back the tears that were burning in my throat. I felt so much in that moment, but anger was in the forefront. Once I got home, I called Laura again to get the number to Dr. Tedishini and made an appointment. I had done a lot of research in the meanwhile and had identified other common culprits that may have been causing her to be sick. While waiting for her appointment, I cut out soy and wheat in addition to the dairy that we'd avoided for most of her life. Nothing seemed to make a difference, but I chose to put my faith in Dr. Tedishini and our upcoming visit. I set aside my own feelings of inadequacy and my frustration with our situation, as the health of Zandra became of much greater significance. I was her advocate and the only person who could be. I was the only person who spent every day with her and knew what she looked like when something wasn't right. I was the one she was honest with when she wanted her own pain to end. I was her mom.

I felt emboldened, and I reflected back to a time when Zandra was only four months old and I had to bring out the warrior mom within me. I had a last-minute opportunity to go to Cuba with my friend, Lina. I had never taken a trip like this before. The price was right and, if I was able to secure a passport in the final hour, I would be off in less than a week. Things lined up for me. Kelley was supportive and knew that as a new mom this adventure would be good for me. These were the kinds of things I thought I had given up as a young mom, but I began to realize that these opportunities could still exist for me. The trip was amazing. I didn't have a beach body, but the sun was therapeutic and, after an adventurous trip to Havana, a lifelong love of history began. It felt truly magical. Walking down ancient streets, seeing old theatres, and walking through palaces and fortresses once seemed like adventures that were for someone else, but now I was living the dream. I had never seen such history and the feeling transcended anything I had ever known. Getting out of the microcosm of my life as a daughter, mother, sister and wife allowed me the opportunity to detach enough to see that there was more outside the confines of my comfort zone.

When I came home from the trip, I was greeted with a sick husband and daughter. Kelley had done well in looking after Zandra and had taken the precaution of taking her to the hospital when she had a fever and showed symptoms of illness. I had no doubt that, as he was also sick, not much sleep was had at home while I was on my dream vacation. The doctor had indicated that Zandra had an ear infection and prescribed her the antibiotic penicillin. I was hospitalized on my ninth birthday with a severe allergy to penicillin, so immediate alarm bells started going off in my head when I heard that Zandra was on it.

Within minutes of being home I set her down on the bed and began to unzip her little purple sleeper. She had massive welts all over her body. I could see that every part of her was covered, down to her little toes. She had swelling in her ankles that I had never seen before. I was worried that soon her throat would start to constrict. I immediately set her in her car seat and drove to the hospital. After a long wait, a locum doctor came and saw to us. He pulled off her sleeper and assessed the swelling and redness. After no more than a minute of looking at her he responded, "I believe these marks to be flea bites. They appear worse at the diaper area, which is where fleas like to hide." I was stunned. I responded, "It's March and it's still cold out with snow on the ground. She hasn't been to the park as she's been sick, and even if she did, she's four months old and doesn't even crawl!" The doctor advised me that since I had been away for the last week, I couldn't speak to where she had been. He was sure these were flea bites and told me that if they weren't gone in a week to come back, but to continue to use the antibiotic, as it's important to continue to stay the course.

I was furious. I drove straight from the Vegreville hospital to the Grey Nuns Hospital in Edmonton with a distressed baby. I was legitimately fearful that she would stop breathing if the swelling reached her throat. Once I had waited through the next set of emergency procedures, I was greeted by another doctor. I explained that I had just come from another hospital and didn't believe that what she had was flea bites. The doctor immediately agreed and scolded me that drug reactions need immediate attention, as if I wasn't the one who had just driven her a panicked hour and a half to get another opinion. He told me that she was experiencing a reaction from the penicillin and wrote me another prescription for her infection. He told me never to give her that antibiotic again, as her ankles were swollen and the next time it could be her throat.

When I left the hospital for the drive home, I was different. I had proven my value that day as a mom and had trusted my instinct even when it opposed one of authority. This step, albeit a small one, provided me with a spark of confidence that sometimes I knew best.

When the day of the appointment arrived with Dr. Tedishini, I was nervous yet ready. Dr. Tedishini was in a new clinic, different from the one that I recalled from being a child, but he was just the same. He was balding a little more, but still spoke with the familiar voice from my childhood. He was delighted to meet my girls and was quick to notice the dark circles and bloated stomach on Zandra. He knew, just like me, that this wasn't normal. We spoke of her medical history; I was careful to remain guarded that he might dismiss her symptoms if they couldn't be proven.

Dr. Tedishini was nothing less than an angel to me on that day. He told me that he believed that food intolerances were real and as dangerous to a child as an allergy. He said that years ago, while living in Toronto with his young family, his wife noticed a similar illness with their daughter. Although tests couldn't prove an allergy, he knew that the child's mother's instinct said more than any medical test. They followed an elimination diet that indicated wheat was of great trouble to her, and once they avoided it she was fine. He described the diet and encouraged me to try it with Zandra. He told me that I was on the right track as I was already eliminating foods and to always trust my gut. He said that Zandra's digestion was weak and would take time to heal before we saw things like bloating and dark circles go away. He told me it could take up to six months and to be patient—he even suggested alternative medicine to help balance her. What he gave me was hope. I left his office that day with the confidence that I knew my child better than anyone and that I had permission to relax, as the throwing up and circles around her eyes wouldn't leave overnight.

Doctor Tedishini was right, it did take six months, but after that time life was much more normal. Zandra proved to be intolerant to milk, wheat and soy products. By this time, Joseph—baby number three—had arrived. Life was much better for Zandra in so many ways, but being different was hard. She turned down attending her first birthday party in preschool because it was a pizza party with ice cream cake. I insisted that I could send her with her own food, but she already felt out of place. She noticed that the kids at school looked at her lunches and commented that it wasn't normal—no cheese strings, puddings and packaged cookies. They noticed her sandwiches were made with dense bread and her cookies were always homemade. She was being teased. In the early 2000s, gluten-, dairy- and soy-free food options weren't mainstream. We had to drive to Edmonton to find her groceries and it never appeared the same as "regular" food. I was getting quite good at making things from scratch, but it deeply bothered her to be different. Things were acceptable within her own home. The Easter Bunny would fill her basket with some of her favourite things: olives, beef jerky and dried fruit and nuts. These were things she always openly loved, but nothing that she saw her peers eating in preschool, or later when she got to elementary. Zandra wanted to fit in with her peers, just as most children do. As much as I encouraged her that being different was courageous and special, she just wanted to be normal.

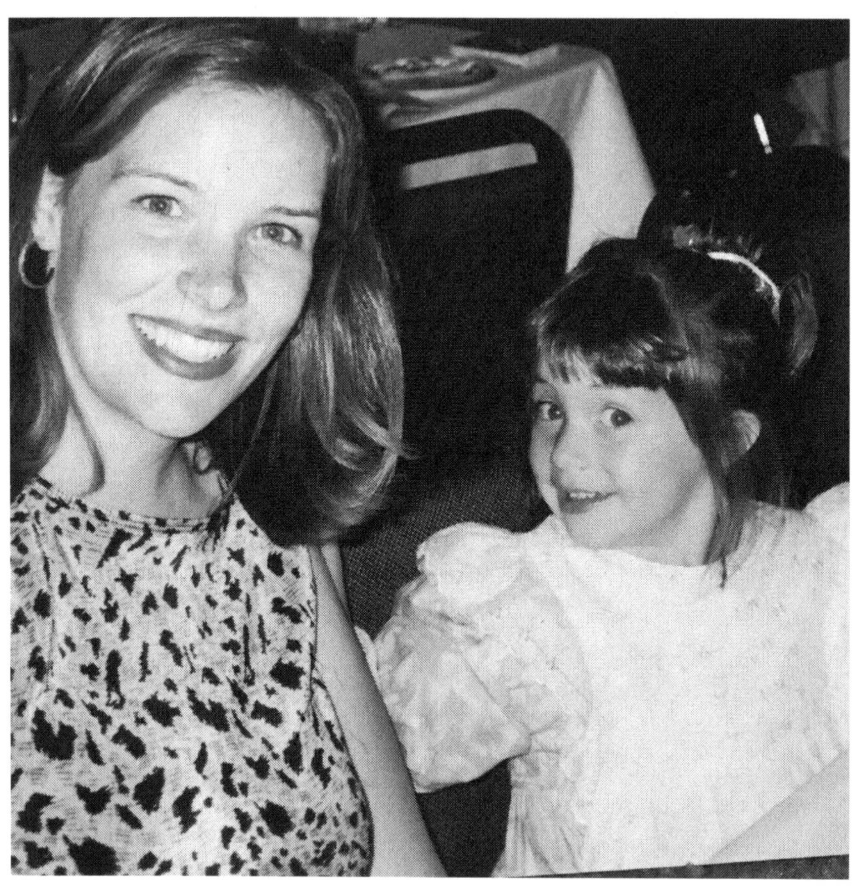

Janet and Zandra in the early years

CHAPTER 3

My Calling

The voice was clear and commanding. It sounded male, yet I couldn't describe it as such. It felt like a father speaking to his child, but it was a voice that, although familiar, wasn't one I could put a name to. I couldn't describe it any other way than to say it spoke through me and above all other ambient sounds. The voice was clear, as if I was underwater, and all the other sounds around me faded into a distant hum and the voice that called me was the only thing that was clear—as if speaking to me directly through headphones. The voice always called my name—Janet—and repeated the call until I acknowledged it. Often I would run upstairs, responding as if it was a call from a parent, knowing full well that it wasn't the familiar sound of my parents' voices. I always erred on the side of caution and either asked my sisters if they heard my name being called or checked with my mom for fear she was cross with me.

The sound of my name being called would at times wake me up from a deep sleep. On these occasions I knew it was a call from somewhere other than a physical voice, but I was unsure whose it was. I once asked my mom whose voice I was hearing. I explained the frequency of the voice and how strange it felt to know my name was being called but not know who was calling. I was trying in earnest to answer the call. Mom replied that it was my guilty conscience. She repeated one of her favourite sayings: "Tell the truth and shame the devil." I was around eight years old and, although I knew I wasn't always pure in thought at all times, I couldn't figure out what I had done that was so bad that I needed to confess. The quest to find my caller consumed a lot of my thoughts at that time and continued for years to come.

At a young age, I realized that I couldn't believe everything my mother told me. My sisters and I were big eavesdroppers. We would often be listening around corners or sitting on the stairs that led down to the basement, careful not to step on the top one that squeaked. We would hear Mom talking endlessly for hours about the things that were wrong in her life. Her capacity to talk on the phone to multiple people and share the same story, verbatim, was a skill that she could have monopolized when she had the opportunity. She often warned us, "Those who listen around corners hear ill of themselves." This proved true yet was too irresistible to pass over. We were bored and she did a lot of talking. The temptation was too much. On many occasions, when it suited her, she would speak about how her girls were talented violinists, not to mention recipients of top academic honours at school. There were four kids in my family: three older girls—all born within a four-year span—and a boy born five years after my younger sister. I was the middle girl. These tales were completely false, woven to apportion credit to my mother for raising such amazing girls (not to mention the extraordinary gene pool that we came from).

Listening to conversations around corners for years not only proved to me that my mother was capable of fabricating stories, it confirmed that I wasn't good enough as I was, that even my own mother needed to lie about me. My mom immigrated to Canada from England as one of the many baby boomers whose families were looking outside of their country for opportunity. My grandfather, who we so affectionately called Gangy (because my older sister wasn't able to pronounce granddad and instead came up with a gibberish term that stuck), fought for his country in the British Navy. He was highly intelligent and creative, as well as sharp-tongued and opinionated. He loved his family and expected everyone to be as disciplined and ambitious as he was. As an adult, I can now understand why my mother felt the need to make up stories of our successes. Our accomplishments reflected on her. Although my mom felt she had the approval of her father, I was now in a position to keep up the lie for her without having to be asked. I didn't want to shame her for her lies and disappoint my grandfather with the truth—that his granddaughter was ordinary. My sisters, although we didn't speak of it, also did their best to play up to the stories that were spun about us.

There was often a lot of in-house entertainment. My older sister, Karen, was the apple of my mom's eye, resembling my mom in a lot of ways, both in personality and appearance. She was outgoing, charismatic and very creative. As she grew, so did her artistic talent, and she was able to paint and draw whatever came to mind. Then there was me, eighteen months later. I was sensitive and stubborn. With light-brown, reddish hair and a generous smattering of freckles, I was the stereotypical middle child. Then came my younger sister Laura, less than two years after me. She was small at birth and, as she grew, she developed Snow White features, including dark hair, light skin and green eyes. School came easily for Laura, although she was deathly shy in groups. Five years after Laura came my brother, the apple of my eye. Michael was the sweetest baby I had ever seen. We had an immediate bond and could understand each other without words. We were as bonded as two siblings could be. Often closer to him than our parents, my sisters and I began to fill in as his caregivers when our home life began to unravel.

Mom would often poke fun at her own mother, whom we knew as Nanna. She became the source of blame for Mom's troubles, whom she considered less intelligent and weaker than her dad. Nanna was a homemaker; making clothes, meals and doing laundry was how she provided for her family. I felt that in my mom's opinion, her choice to provide a stable home life and become a support for her family was viewed as feeble and one that received little respect.

Mom and her younger sisters, Vicky and Ginny, all encouraged and pursued rewarding careers. My mom, Dawn, was a psychiatric nurse before the demons in her life took over full time. With a sharp mind, a heart of giving and a flair for the dramatic, this was a great vocation for her. My sisters and I would often call her Elizabeth Taylor, as she had what we called an old-Hollywood personality. Mom had a highly addictive disposition, and from what we knew of the classic stars, they all too often found themselves wrapped up in their own addictions. One of Mom's favourite sayings, "She has to be the bride at every wedding and the corpse at every funeral," spoke to her own personality the most.

Vicky, Mom's younger sister by four years, became a teacher, and then went back to university to pursue a law degree, eventually owning her own business. Ginny was eleven years younger than her. She pursued a career as a respiratory therapist and progressed into management within the health department. With who I considered at the time strong female role models, I knew that my choice was polarized. I could become soft like my Nanna and choose to stay at home and raise my children, or strong like my grandfather, mom and aunties and pursue a career. My dad went to work after high school, working his way up the ranks through a building supply company. His choice of career was criticized by Mom, who felt superior for having graduated post-secondary and earned a higher wage than him. Although she didn't say it, she often implied that she married below her station.

I felt incongruence within myself. I didn't know what I wanted, but I knew how I wanted to be perceived and I felt a strong desire to be respected. I decided that things could be broken down into simple black and white terms, yet I felt strong and weak, loving and harsh, and didn't see a place for me in the world. I couldn't simplify my feelings enough to understand myself.

From my earliest memories I watched the World Vision programs on TV, exposing the suffering that was most often ignored around the globe. I would watch the video coverage of the starving children who seemed utterly unphased by the flies buzzing around their faces. I was also drawn into the shows that depicted orphaned elephants mourning while their mothers lay dead beside them, murdered for their ivory. I couldn't reconcile the type of humans that allowed this type of pain to exist around them with the people I knew in my life. My heart ached and I would sit and cry, compelled to watch and wonder how I could help. I watched these programs in secret, continuing well into adulthood. I felt as though I was being called to a higher purpose, as if a voice was speaking right to me. It was often when I was watching these programs that I heard the call of my name.

When I was young, I would daydream of healing. Most often I saw myself as a veterinarian who would go into places like Africa to set up elephant sanctuaries and help in the villages that needed it. I would see myself in khaki pants and a white linen button-up shirt. I would satisfy my heart's desire with these fantasies, including myself as a beautiful woman with a handsome husband and a wallet to match the size of my heart. I never wanted or saw myself with children. Even as a girl, I knew that if my heart could ache for the children of Africa, having my own would overwhelm me.

Nanna was highly spiritual and a loving follower of Christ. She would turn to scripture to help her solve her problems and would occasionally speak in tongues at church or at home. I resented her for her softness as I grew, assuming my mom's perspective, even though my resentment was only ever matched with love and acceptance. Nanna was quiet when the world got noisy and gentle when the world was harsh, and used humour when the world was too serious. She never lost her patience with me. She saw me through the lens of love and I never appreciated her until after she was gone. I am grateful now more than ever for her presence in my life, and allow her to be a part of my heart by seeing things through her eyes as often as I can. Nanna loved all creatures, especially birds and rabbits. She loved her British shows and we often shared laughs over her favourite, *All Creatures Great and Small.* Nanna loved her garden, her Bible and her animals. I too enjoy these things now and celebrate the little humorous things that happen in life. I still feel comforted by the sound of an English accent and words such as "blimey" and "bonnie lass." I think if I had asked Nanna about the voice that called my name, I would have heard a much different answer than I got from Mom. Perhaps that answer would have filled me with love and purpose. But I was meant to take a path that took me into the depths of my soul, to where understanding, forgiveness and purpose are born.

As the years passed, I would continue to hear my name in the familiar call. It became a comfort to me. Hearing my name, even when I knew I was in a room or the house by myself, told me that I wasn't alone. Someone or something out there knew me. Even when hearing my name became less frequent, the knowledge that I was visible became the crutch that would get me through years of loneliness that my younger self had no idea would come.

The first prayer I can recall praying was around age five. I asked God to make me special. Specifically, I wanted to be a prodigy, much like Mom led people to believe I was, although it wasn't the truth. It didn't matter to me what my gift was, just that I had one. I'm not sure why I requested such a thing from God at such a young age. Perhaps it originated from my faith, having been brought up in the Anglican Church believing that everyone was created for a purpose, and I was eager to know my own reason for being. Or maybe it came from deep insecurities that were present from early on, believing that in order to be worthy, I had to be special.

This prayer became a perpetual request, followed by the disappointment that in every way I was proving to be ordinary. As I got older, I realized that my time to become a prodigy was running out. I felt as though I had to prove my value to my family before I was lost in a barren wasteland of underachievers. In a family where praise and acceptance were earned by achievement, I was proving to be a disappointment. I felt undeserving of the food on my plate and the clothes on my back. I struggled to accept gifts on my birthday, feeling completely unworthy of the time and effort put into acknowledging me. My mom continually reminded me there were children all over the world who were more deserving than my sisters and me, and yet they lived in poverty with disease and war around them and I was spared. I believed deep in my heart that God had a purpose and plan for me, yet the older I got, the more critical my inner dialogue became. I found myself lost in the belief that there was no value in being ordinary, a lie I believed for far too long.

It would take me many years to understand that an ordinary emotion such as empathy was indeed an extraordinary gift. I could feel the emotions of others so deeply and on the same level as my own. I realized that I was different in this way. When friends could laugh at the expense of another, I never could, even as a joke. If I did, I was torn up about it inside to the point I felt ill. I was able to look at a photo and feel the mood in myself. I could walk into a room and know what others were feeling, yet there was no language to understand or express myself. These feelings further isolated me from others. I wasn't able to be as carefree as I saw others were. I lost myself in the confusion of emotions within my home, school and outside world. I couldn't separate my own feelings of despair from those I felt around me. I found it impossible to feel happy when I felt that others were not, and as I grew I became a sort of chameleon. Without effort, I knew what was needed. I could fill the gaps and be fun and spontaneous or a quiet listener for whomever needed me. At the best of times I felt I had a purpose and was needed, and at the worst of times I felt disconnected and out of tune with my own feelings.

In a house where my parents struggled with mental illness and addiction, the conditions grew toxic with every passing year. Overwhelming emotions developed within me and, as much as I contorted myself to be what my parents expected and needed, I was unable to heal the gaping wounds that were hemorrhaging around me. My world felt unstable and unpredictable.

I learned quickly that being alone replenished my soul. I felt connected to a source that was invisible to me, yet somehow revitalized me. Conversely, I learned that being around others easily depleted my happiness, especially when they were sad, jealous and anxious. There was no hiding it from me—I always knew.

The first ten years of my life felt idyllic. I had parents with stable jobs and an extended family whom I felt close to. I felt as if my home was a modern-day *Little House on the Prairie*. Sure we had struggles, but so did the Ingalls. As I grew older, so did the tensions within my parents' relationship. I knew my dad had a difficult childhood. He lost his father unexpectedly at age two and then his beloved stepfather around age ten, and when his mom remarried for a third time, the new husband proved to be cruel and abusive. Dad had to drop out of high school to support his other five siblings, as well as his mother, to get away from the abuse and death threats. Mom had her own set of traumas. Following WWII, Mom's parents left the UK for Canada seeking a better life with their young family. Her parents struggled to put the past behind them. My grandfather would often drink, and he confessed late in life how hard he was on his girls. From my own observations, and later family confirmations, I could see my mom struggle with bulimia, borderline personality disorder and bipolar disorder. The combination of my parents' traumas created a lot of distress and angst within the family home. I always felt grateful that for the first years of my life I felt supported, yet sadly that wasn't the case for my brother.

In our house, alone time was scarce, so when I got older and people needed house sitters to look after their pets while on holidays, I was the first to volunteer. For me, animals were always different—they never wore me down. Although I could pick up on their emotions, they didn't drain me in the same way people did. My animals were very much my best friends throughout my childhood and the path by which I could escape the overwhelming world of people.

I was especially close with our two Siamese cats: Alphie and Percy. These two souls were, without a doubt, sent by God. Whenever myself or one of my siblings was sick, lonely or upset, the cats wouldn't leave us alone for a minute, not even to eat. They were angels in the form of cats for me, solidifying my trust of animals to this day. Percy was the best alarm clock. He would come down to my room in the basement to wake me up every morning. When I wouldn't wake easily, he would carefully grab my eyelashes with his teeth and pull my eyelids open. I would usually smell his cat breath and sense his presence before I felt my eyes being opened. We also had a dog, Taffy. She was a little terrier cross with soft, blond fur and bent little ears. She was very much my mom's beloved pet, following her around the house room to room, always sitting at her feet, closer to her than any of her own children ever could be. The jealousy that I felt when Taffy won Mom's affections hardened my heart to her, and she became the only animal I disliked, but this changed near the end of her life.

When I was eight years old, Taffy became sick. I was unaware because of my age of the symptoms that brought her to the veterinarian, but I was fully present and aware of the diabetes diagnosis that she was given. The only other time I heard of diabetes was being told that great-nanna in England had diabetes and that's why she became blind. I was told that great-nanna had beautiful violet eyes, admired by everyone who saw her, and diabetes tragically took away her greatest asset. I didn't understand at the time what diabetes was but was told that her body didn't produce enough insulin for some reason, and that she needed injections to compensate at mealtimes. I was quick to volunteer for the job of helping Taffy. Mom was always someone I looked up to, even when she was cruel. She had beautiful black hair, brown eyes, olive skin and a petite figure. In our house, her nursing background meant that things like doctor's visits and needles were no big deal. They were all parts of what Mom dealt with daily at work. Having a nurse in the house always gave me great comfort as a child. I always knew that Mom could help in an emergency and felt that Taffy couldn't be in a better home with her disease.

Mom taught me to keep the insulin in the refrigerator to preserve it. She showed me how to draw the insulin into the needle, pinch a spot on Taffy's back and inject it slowly while she was eating and unaware. It was an easy job that gave me great satisfaction. It also helped my hardened heart to soften, seeing her so vulnerable and needing me when Mom was at work or away. I could never say that I grew close with Taffy, but once my walls came down I began to feel her emotions. She started to follow me around, just like she did Mom. I could feel that she had a big heart that trusted me.

I knew Taffy was a stray and had found her way to us, but until then I didn't feel her love for myself. Instead, I had allowed my jealousy to act as a shield, not allowing myself to feel at all. I supported a very black and white perspective when I couldn't manage my own emotions. I became polarized in my perspectives. I either loved or hated, agreed or disagreed, cared or didn't care—this attitude led to my label of the stubborn one.

Taffy lived for several years with diabetes. We were watchful of her food and never missed her insulin. Perhaps we were all too comfortable, because when we left to go to my Nanna's house for supper one Sunday, Taffy got into the Easter chocolate that mom had hidden away under her bed for Easter the following week. Taffy wasn't a big dog, around fifteen pounds, but she managed to get into all four of the one-pound bunnies. By the time we got home, her skin had turned blue and was very visible under her nearly transparent blond fur. Taffy was immediately taken to the vet hospital, but despite all that they tried to do for her, she didn't have more than a couple weeks with us after that.

Taffy's health declined greatly in the coming days, and on what we knew would be her last night with us, she came downstairs to my bedroom and stood at my bed. I picked up her ballooned and fragile body and placed her in bed with me. Usually she would be with Mom, but this night, much to my surprise, it was me she wanted. I could see and feel that she was in pain despite the pain medications she was given. I couldn't understand why Taffy wanted me, not Mom as she usually did. What I began to realize was that Taffy was there in Grace. She kept by my side as I wept and apologized for how I had teased her through the years. I would tease her that Nanna, her "second favourite person in the world," was at the door. Taffy would race to the door in excitement and I would tell her, "No, back door." Taffy would then race to the back door to see Nanna. I would go on and on until Taffy submitted in exhaustion, realizing that Nanna wasn't coming. I did this in fun, yet knew it wasn't right. On this last night, I regretted how had I treated her. Just like the cats, she ended up staying by my side for me, not for her. I needed to unburden my heart and she, like an angel with fur, was there to help me, and no matter how horrible I was she forgave me.

Taffy was the first loss I had ever known. At age ten I had no idea that within that decade I would lose my remaining grandparents; the cats; our next family dog, Suzie; and my dad. Taffy's death taught me that I would live through the grief. I would set up a framework that would create a pathway to navigate a broken heart, even if I was doing so on autopilot.

Diabetes never came up in my world again until I met my first boyfriend, Danny. I met Danny in junior high. He was tall with a great sense of humour. I was unaware that he was diabetic at first; he played numerous sports and didn't seem different from anyone else. When we began to date, we would often head to the community basketball courts for hours, playing into the summer days in full heat and exhaustion. Even then I was oblivious to him eating candy or testing. He made his disease look so normal and left me with the impression that there was nothing he couldn't do. At mealtimes he was often discrete with his injections. Sometimes he would make an injection into his stomach, much the same way I did for Taffy: grabbing a pinch of skin and carefully poking the needle into it, then slowly pushing down the plunger of the syringe until all the insulin was gone. Danny's friends were no strangers to seeing him do his injections. I had never seen any situation where he was in jeopardy or not looking after himself.

As we got to high school, I learned that one of my classmates, Greg, had a brother who was also a type 1 diabetic. His name was Aaron and he clearly wasn't taking good care of himself. He was a couple of years older than us and had been experimenting with alcohol. He seemed to be in denial about his condition and would often not take his injections at all. I had been to a couple of house parties at Greg's house and had seen for myself how dismissive Aaron was to his diabetes. Danny's mom, Jean, had warned me that a diabetic low looks a lot like being drunk. She often asked me to watch out for Danny, as she was no doubt nervous about the upcoming experimental phase we were heading into. I rarely drank a drop during my teens. I was happy to look out for my boyfriend, as it gave me an easy excuse to not drink myself. What I didn't tell anyone, not even Danny, was that I wanted nothing to do with anything that could lead to addiction. I lived with my mom's addiction to prescription medication and was living a secret life, hiding not only her addictions but her mental illnesses as well. I felt that I needed to keep control of my own life, and anything that could jeopardize my ability to maintain control was out of the question, even a drink at a party.

Danny told me that refusing to take care of yourself was a sure way to be blind in a short time, as well as exposing yourself to a full host of other conditions, including death. It seemed that he knew of the dark side of diabetes, but as he clearly looked after himself, to me it was a simple choice. If you looked after yourself, nothing could go wrong. Taking care was simply testing blood sugars and injecting insulin. It wasn't until years later when we were no longer together that I heard about his struggles and close calls from the disease.

After high school, I took a year off to work. I had a full-time job at a small engine-repair supply shop that sold parts for lawnmowers, chainsaws and other small-engine machines. I wasn't happy with the work, but it granted me the ability to live independently and, coupled with of my frugal lifestyle, save a decent amount of money.

There were numerous struggles in my house that made living at home impossible for me. I moved away earlier than any of my friends and had a place of my own. My little apartment was everything I needed. I had peace and calm, yet the years of being raised in a home with addiction and mental health created an anxiety that became a constant within me. The shame, grief and turmoil had me feeling unlovable and undeserving. I ended my relationship with Danny and started one with a guy named Kelley, whom I met through a friend.

Kelley didn't have a lot of expectations for the future, and in turn placed none on me. The relationship matched the beliefs I held for myself at the time. I felt like a disappointment to everyone. I didn't know how to survive the mounding stress that was ruminating through my mind and the emotions from other people I hurt. I dealt with relationships by simply cutting them off. I couldn't manage my own pain as well as the pain of anyone else, so I simply disconnected them from my life. My life with Kelley remedied the loneliness I had for a companion and allowed me to feel special. Being in a new relationship placed me on level ground. I felt no expectations or presumptions of where I was or who I should be.

The problems with my mom's addictions and mental health existed, but in my little apartment I could find moments of peace. The year I took to work and save money before going back to school helped me to stand away from the fire I felt from my family. I didn't have the ability to be introspective as I was still in a state of panic and stress, but it was a welcome reprieve from what I had known for the last many years of my life. I managed to graduate in urban and regional planning, and although I really enjoyed the area of study, I was unable to see a future for myself beyond graduation.

I was still in a relationship with Kelley when my dad died by suicide. It happened shortly after my graduation, on Halloween, and left me in a world of pain. My family was hurting, and that Christmas, while away for the holidays, a family friend mentioned that we should start planning my wedding. I had been engaged but had wanted to extend my engagement a couple of years to see how I really felt about marriage. Instead, I found myself in full planning mode, creating something that would pull everyone together in a celebration to look forward to. I desperately wanted a purpose. I was stuck in my grief like a fly in a web, and the planners around me gave me a reason to get unstuck. If I had listened to my heart, I would have heard that it was telling me to wait, urging me to reconsider. But I had no words. I felt hollow. We were married the following May in 1998.

CHAPTER 4

A New Normal

I'M NOT SURE WHAT I should have expected, whether a doctor would provide us with information, or perhaps a nurse, but nobody came to tell us what to expect, other than we would be told more at the Stollery Children's Hospital in Edmonton. All I had was my own history and the Google search engine on my iPhone. In the meanwhile, the hospital staff would provide insulin by injection and manage Zandra's blood sugars through the emergency doctors in Edmonton until we were able to leave. Zandra was full of questions and understandably scared. I did my best to assure her that diabetes was a common disease and, from what I knew, was quite manageable. After all, Danny lived a full and normal life with the disease—all it would take was extra care. During the night I researched actors with diabetes. We discovered that Halle Berry and Nick Jonas were also diabetic. I assured Zandra that God didn't give us anything we couldn't handle, although I couldn't imagine why any child would be diagnosed with such a life sentence.

We also Googled the University of Alberta Hospital, which was affiliated with the Stollery Children's Hospital, and saw how they were leading the world with diabetes research, even discovering a new and promising treatment: islet cell transplants. We learned that with this transplant doctors were able to transfer islet cells from a donor pancreas into a patient with diabetes so that they could produce insulin and either reduce or eliminate the need for injections.

When we researched the national diabetes association, Diabetes Canada, we saw that lots of people choose to participate in running events across the world to promote awareness and help with research that will eventually lead to a cure. We saw that one of the runs was in Iceland and mused about how we would create our opportunity to go just because of her diabetes. It was very overwhelming for an eleven-year-old, but I did my best to stay optimistic. Inside, I was in panic. My heart was racing, listing all the scenarios that I could imagine lay ahead.

I had to tell Kelley about her diagnosis. It gave me no satisfaction to be right. He was apologetic for his comments and tried to explain that he was only trying to do the right thing. This was my second apology of the day. I forgave both offenders and only thanked God for listening to my inner voice despite all that stood in my way.

The next day, after a long night together in the hospital, we drove to Edmonton to the diabetes clinic at the Stollery. I was scared just being alone with her. It felt like when I was bringing her home as a newborn. What if she stops breathing? What if she needs something and I don't know what to do? I felt completely unsure and so did Zandra. She was scared and I had no way to really relate. My perspective was as her mom, and although the pain was shared, the experience was completely different. Things that I would normally fret about, such as where the clinic was within the hospital or where to park, were of no consequence. I summoned the qualities she would need to lean on. Open-mindedness needed to blend with a carefree spirit and a responsible attitude. It was a challenge for me, yet I had to lead by example.

Going into the hospital I had no idea what was coming our way. I expected her to be admitted into the hospital until we got her stable and learned what to expect. But that wasn't the way it was. We were told that we would meet every day for the week in a class-type setting with her nurse, caregivers and of course Zandra. We were to gather our team and begin right away so we were all on the same page and understood the same information. Our overall commute was almost three hours a day; however, I knew we were lucky. Many families had to stay in a hotel at their own expense or travel much greater distances than us. I called Kelley and he cleared his schedule. He brought his girlfriend,

Carmen, for a couple of days of the training. It was hard for me to be there and form this loving team when I had to fight so hard to get her to the hospital in the first place. The energy it took to make peace and try to trust Kelley to be a safe person for Zandra robbed me of the energy I needed to be present when I needed to be.

The first day provided us all an opportunity to talk to the nurses about the reality of the diagnosis. The very first question that Zandra asked the nurse was whether she could drink alcohol! The question shocked me and amused the nurse. I had never spoken to her about alcohol consumption before, rather leaving her understanding to be demonstrated by our example of drinking on occasion in moderation. Alcohol was never a focus in our family, so the question was a surprise to me. The nurse assured Zandra that her questions were welcome and that this was a natural question for a girl of eleven who was knocking on the door of her teen years. She provided professional and accurate information about how alcohol lowers blood sugars, so mixing it in a drink with juice could offset the effects. She spoke of how the effects of alcohol and low blood sugar are strikingly similar and that many people get into trouble because they are left alone to "sleep it off," when in fact they need sugar in a desperate way. Zandra followed that question with another equally surprising question: "Will I be able to have children?" This was something I had never imagined her thinking about. Again, the nurse answered her thoughtful question, assuring her that every day diabetic women have healthy babies without any problems.

The rest of the day included very strict calculations of every type of food that she ate. She had a regimented meal, which was balanced out by the nutritionist. Every item, whether it was a carbohydrate or vegetable, had to be weighed and calculated. This system was called "multiple daily injections," or MDI. She would always calculate what they called "carbs" for her food ahead of time and how much insulin she would need for it, offset by her existing blood sugar. But to begin, we needed to stabilize her until she didn't have ketones and got the hang of things.

Ketones, we were told, are chemicals that the body creates when it breaks down fat to use for energy. The body does this when it doesn't have insulin to use the sugar, which is the body's normal energy source. When ketones build up in the blood you can develop DKA, which is "diabetic ketoacidosis." This condition is extremely dangerous and can happen quickly for a type 1 diabetic. The extreme thirst and frequent urination were the signs that Zandra was already in DKA. We had to combat this with measured insulin and copious amounts of water.

After the first day, I was sent home with Zandra from the hospital with a binder full of information about diabetes and her diet plan, as well as charts of what were called "carb ratios"—a quick way to multiply the weight of the food with its carb ratio to determine the total carbs of the food. We were set up with a homecare nurse to help with the injections for the first couple of days, until we felt confident doing it ourselves. Since the first day of her diagnosis, Zandra didn't want anyone giving her the injection. She decided with bull-headed determination that she would be in control. She refused to give me or anyone else a part to play in her care.

The practical planning of taking myself out of my daily household role to attend these classes was a challenge. Gord asked his mom to come for the week and she graciously drove the three and a half hours from her hometown of Wandering River to take over. Knowing that Liam was cared for was a huge burden taken from me. Gord was able to arrange his schedule to attend a couple of days of training; however, his court schedule, which was booked many months in advance, didn't allow him to be present for all of the training days. Kelley was able to clear his schedule for the week and so was Carmen, something that made Zandra very happy. Olivia and Joseph were still with Kelley and all of the information about Zandra would be explained through them. I felt strongly that they would benefit by staying with Zandra at my house throughout this training so they could physically see her and be assured that, although Zandra was sick, she would ultimately be okay. As we left to go home in the afternoons, there would be plenty of time for Zandra to spend time with them, and as siblings so often communicate, they wouldn't even need to talk to gain comfort from each other's presence and feel assured. I knew Olivia and Joseph would be concerned for her and I felt Zandra would benefit in having her siblings around to confide in, but Kelley didn't want me having them. I wanted to fight to have them stay with me so that they could be with my mother-in-law and Liam in the day and Zandra at night, but I didn't have the fight in me. Kelley didn't want to relinquish his week, and instead made arrangements to have them placed with various friends while he and Carmen attended the classes. I had to trust God to comfort and ease their worries until I saw them again that Friday night. Although they were young, I felt they were denied the opportunity to support their sister and understand what was happening. Diabetes, like most diseases, affects the entire family, not just the one diagnosed.

Coming home was scary for both of us. On our way, Zandra and I stopped at the Safeway grocery store, which was only a couple of blocks from the hospital, so we would have a sugar snack on hand for emergency low blood sugar. We found that everything that was quick and convenient was filled with preservatives and other additives, like artificial colour and flavour. We quickly became seasoned label readers, and before long knew how many carbs were in servings of food by memory and what was healthy versus what was *labelled* healthy. We settled on packaged cookies and juice boxes.

In addition to the new diet regimen, we had to do blood sugar checks throughout the night, once at midnight and once at two a.m. I had learned how to use the glucose monitor at the hospital, replacing the tiny needle to prick the finger and using the test strips that the blood drop touched. Zandra's bedroom was in the basement of our two-storey house. We had developed the basement just before Liam was born to provide space for each child to have their own bedroom. Zandra and Liv never successfully shared a room; as a true older sister, Zandra tormented Liv to tears on more than one occasion. Her new room had beautiful walnut furniture and two-toned purple walls to match the queen-sized bedding that we bought for her. Her room was beautiful. I would have loved it for myself. Now the distance that once created harmony within our household felt like vast worlds apart. I wouldn't be able to hear her call out in the night if she needed help. I wasn't sure that she should have to travel so far to access help or sugar if she needed it. I took the baby monitor from Liam's room and used it as a way for Zandra to call out in the night should she need me. She felt this was a huge violation of her privacy and rarely turned it on. I was scared and found myself awake through the night, listening out as if I had a newborn in the house again, except this time it would be a definite distress call, not a diaper change or hunger.

At least twice a night for several months, I would travel up and down two flights of stairs to test for blood sugars, and more often just to listen and watch for the gentle rising and falling of her breath under the covers. This nighttime routine became such a burden that we sold our house and moved into one where all of the bedrooms could be on the same floor. This move eased my worries and made nighttime checks much less of an ordeal.

I wasn't very good at testing, so it wasn't long before Zandra took over the nighttime tests on her own, with me only coming to her room and acting as a reminder and a backup source of knowledge for how to manage the blood sugar results. She wanted to eliminate my presence all together, but I knew that she needed me when she woke up groggy and wasn't confident how to proceed. Although she tried to shut me out, I remained firm in my presence by her bedside.

The first homecare nurse who came to the house just happened to be someone we both knew. Her name was Sandra, and her son was in the 4H group that Zandra had been in a year earlier. We had been out to their farm for the dog-agility portion of the program, bringing with us our dear Murphy. Sandra was a kind, consoling woman who shared firsthand knowledge of diabetes, as her husband was also diabetic. Having Sandra come was a godsend to both Zandra and me. She was professional yet personable and knew our family. She was genuinely sympathetic toward Zandra's disease, yet optimistic in her outlook for a full and healthy life. I felt as though I needed the comforting and encouraging more than Zandra.

We only needed the health nurse for a couple of days before Zandra was able to administer her own needles, and we had the comfort of an on-call nurse twenty-four hours a day. We had regular appointments at the hospital for regular check-ins once the weeklong class was over. We would see the doctor, dietician and a social worker. Each member of this team was tasked with making sure that patients were cared for and supported, both physically and emotionally. From the beginning, it was clear that Zandra was angry. She had a chip on her shoulder that sent the message that she alone was the one who was suffering. When anything was mentioned about my concerns, she was quick to clear up the confusion that it was her disease and her burden, not mine.

During these appointments it often felt as though Zandra was throwing me under the bus. She would find fault with something I did or didn't do and make a point of letting the doctor and other professionals know it. Despite all the advocating, research and work I would put toward her care, she would find a way to take her personal frustration out against me in this public way. This seemed to happen time after time, appointment after appointment.

At first I felt humiliated, and angry toward her. I would question her after the appointment and let her know how I felt. She was ruthless in her conviction and didn't back down. It appeared as though she could turn her anger on and off, like a lever that needed to release every now and again. These appointments served as a vent for her pent-up anger, and the more positive affirmation she got from the doctors that she was managing things well, the more she would turn on me. At first, I felt like I needed to tell the truth and let them know that I was following her records and harping on her to record her blood sugars. I would try to assert that I was measuring her food for her in her lunch when she didn't think I was. Eventually I decided that they likely saw the truth, although they didn't say as much. They were careful to demonstrate that they were on Team Zandra, her ally and supporter. I was grateful for their approach, yet I needed a boost. I too felt alone, hurt and angry. I wondered why my daughter struggled, and why she had lost the carefree innocence that all children deserve. I felt as though I needed the same type of reassurance that she received. I was frustrated that a job well done for me meant that she would be alive to see another day, and all the agony that was felt in the long days and nights was felt silently, without witness.

In the beginning we were both keen to keep accurate records and have clear information for the doctors to make their adjustments; however, that dedication waned within the first year. The doctors assured us that this was normal preteen behaviour, but they were quick to warn us that it was dangerous. On a couple of occasions, we learned that our appointments were delayed because one of the other patients had passed away. It was a real-life danger that every now and again reminded us that although diabetes was manageable, it was dangerous with no real cure.

CHAPTER 5

Moving Forward

After Kelley and I separated, I wanted someone who really saw me for all that I lived and hoped for. I wanted a partner who wouldn't settle, someone who wanted to make a difference in this world and wasn't afraid of obstacles. When I finally started seeing that those qualities existed in me, I found someone who mirrored that in my own life.

I met Gord several years prior to our relationship. His sister Sheryl was the operator of the day home that Zandra went to, and she and I had become fast friends. Sheryl had energy for life like nobody I had ever met. She saw opportunities and seized upon them fearlessly. She had an edge that I was sure could bite, but she brought out my own fearlessness and determination. Her brother was younger than her by ten years, closer to my age. He was in law school and engaged when I met him the first time. At that time, I was pregnant with Olivia and didn't think of him as anything other than my friend's brother. He had dark brown/black hair that was coming in white at an early age. I had kept in the loop with his life through his sister, even hearing about the breakup of his relationship. Gord had decided to take a transfer within the Crown prosecutor's office where he worked to be closer to his sister and her family. It wasn't until then that I got to actually know him. He was one of the most introspective and thoughtful men I had ever met. He saw me in a way that was refreshing to me. I felt safe around him; I could let my guard down, let him know my strengths and weaknesses, and he would only ever see me as perfect.

The timing of my relationship was concerning for us and for everyone around us. I had separated from Kelley after Joseph was born. The problems in our marriage had become overwhelming and, after trying for years, I didn't see a happy future for myself. I knew that a heart took time to heal and that rebounding was harmful, especially when there are kids. I knew all of this yet felt a magnetic charge so powerful that I knew Gord was meant for me. I judged myself harshly. I closed myself off from everyone who saw me as I did, yet I knew deep down I was on the right track. I knew my children would feel as though I had just replaced their dad. They were too young to know that my heart had been out of my marriage for so long that although the timing seemed sudden, it was not. I had played into the appearances of a happy marriage for so long that I had fooled nearly everyone who knew me, and sometimes myself. This wasn't sudden at all. I had the daunting task of forgiving myself.

They say forgiveness is a decision you make. Every day I had to pledge to love and forgive myself. I now had to change my heart so that I earned my own respect and loved myself unconditionally. My decision to maintain a relationship with Gord cost me friends and family. It was the most difficult crossroads to be in and I felt the kind of despair that I'm sure my dad felt when he made the decision to leave this world. If it weren't for knowing firsthand the pain of losing a parent to suicide, I fear my mind would have surely wandered down that lonely path. My children saved me from losing the opportunity to know and love myself, even if at the time they were hurt and angry. Despite what the previous day brought, I made a fresh decision each morning to forgive and move forward. I also promised myself that whatever the kids may feel toward me, I would be there for them. They needed me, and even though they likely wouldn't realize it for many years, I knew that when they became parents themselves I would be there for them.

Despite the strained relationships within the family, Gord and I knew that we were stronger together. We were each other's best friend and supporter. We both knew that the kind of love we shared was magical and could heal the world, starting with ourselves. We were married on October 3, 2009, the day after my thirty-third birthday. We married in his family church, which was a small country church seating about forty people. It had no power or gas, so it was heated with a wood stove and lit by the natural light of the windows and candles. We had beautiful fresh arrangements of seasonal autumn flowers, and the girls and I wore simple off-white dresses. During the wedding ceremony, there were hundreds of monarch butterflies surrounding the little candlelit church as if they were attendees waiting to catch a glimpse through the windows. The ceremony was the most special wedding I have ever seen. Joseph, who was only four years old, walked me down the aisle. When the minister asked him if he would give me away, he answered, "I won't give her away, but I'll share her." The memory of those words still brings a tear to my eye and a smile to my face.

Prior to our wedding, Gord and I spoke of having more children. Having babies was hard on my body, both in pregnancy and delivery. With all of the pregnancies I had experienced high blood pressure and severe edema, as well as hemorrhaging after the birth of my last two. Gord had expressed that although he always wanted children, he never felt he needed his own. He was happy to be a stepdad, as he loved the kids immensely. Something in me wanted another baby. I was afraid that wanting another child was a default setting within me, wanting to take care of others and knowing that having a child was a long commitment to do just that. I didn't want to cut myself short and delay other dreams for the safe decision to have a child, so the decision weighed heavily on my mind. The decision to have a baby began to build up pressure and immediacy. There was no explanation for it; we were engaged but not married; we had a lot of time to decide to grow a family.

Often when I need to make a decision I go out in nature. I knew that I needed to make a big one, so I set out with a backpack and supplies for the day. I grabbed Murphy and headed out into the valley, not to return until I had connected with the part of me that knew my heart's answer. I didn't let anyone in on the purpose of my hike; these types of walks were so personal, between my spirit, God and, always, Murphy. On this walk, I hiked until my body was exhausted. My thoughts were given the space to go from the mundane distractions of *What's for supper?* to *Do I like my hair colour?* until I bravely asked what my thoughts were about having a baby. I sat on the trail with Murphy panting under my arm and waited for the answer that I knew would come. The answer was *Yes, and soon*. The urgency surprised me, but I was learning to trust what came to me. Gord was supportive of the decision that would greatly impact both our lives, although I felt reluctant to reveal the process of how the answer came to me. By the time of our wedding I was in the first trimester.

The pregnancy was healthy, but by no means easy. Zandra was angry with me. She reacted to the pregnancy by telling me, "You're ruining my life!" She dreamt of life going back to the way it used to be before the divorce, and now this made her dream a little more impossible. I was also sure that she anticipated her dad's reaction and took on the role of his voice and advocate. Olivia and Joseph were happy and excited in equal measure to meet their new sibling.

About a month after the wedding, Gord began experiencing a lot of pain in his knee. He was in the beginning of a first-degree murder trial and with that came a lot of pressure. He didn't have time for the inconvenience and the growing pain was making it harder to do his job. At the beginning of the weeklong trial, his knee was making it hard to stand in the courtroom, and by the end he simply couldn't. He had to request special permission not to rise when the judge entered the court. This pain didn't let up after the trial. It intensified, making it almost impossible to sleep, and it began to move: one night his knee, the next his shoulder, the next his ankle. When the pain was in the joint it felt as if it was burning and broken, he could swear that it was, although he didn't know of a cause. After several trips to the doctor and a battery of blood tests, Gord was diagnosed with rheumatoid arthritis. This was the same disease that I had seen ravage my Nanna and Mom. I didn't know life without it, and it seemed that I never would. My heart sank into a grief that Gord thankfully didn't understand. He didn't know what he was in for, he only knew that life was increasingly difficult. He couldn't even walk into the doctor's office without my arm for support. He often couldn't tie his tie or shoes. He couldn't shift the gears in his car or hold his boxes of files. Gord was given a series of medications to try, and meanwhile I was his pregnant caretaker.

When Gord was first prescribed methotrexate, an immune system suppressant, he was warned that if we wanted to have children it was important that he not be on the medication, as it could result in serious problems with the fetus. I now understood the immediacy of my pregnancy. I was grateful for the spiritual nudge in making a swift decision. I no longer questioned my own agenda in understanding the feelings and vowed to provide space in future when God has a plan for me. Gord would often joke: "It's a good thing I got the 'sickness and health' vows in before the diagnosis!"

When Liam was born, the medication Gord was on had finally started to work. Gord didn't yet feel secure in holding Liam, but at least he could sit with him. I felt so grateful that something was moving in the right direction. It had been a long haul to get to where we were, and I was feeling full in spirit but exhausted in body. Liam was a fussy baby. He reminded me a lot of Zandra, not only in looks but personality. Both babies didn't seem to want or need sleep and were highly demanding. They were both brunettes with wide, blue eyes. This was my chance to parent differently. This was my chance to heal my family by example. I hoped that I could demonstrate a transformed part of me through raising Liam, a part that would bring us closer together.

Zandra wasn't doing well. She was even more distraught than what I expected from a normal, jealous sibling and surpassed what I thought would be a reasonable transition time. Zandra was beyond upset, so I had taken her to the doctor and he decided to start investigating with a blood test. He was thorough in his investigation, and days later his office called with the results. Everything was normal except for her vitamin D levels—apparently they were severely low. Most people's are considered low, especially for those living in the northern hemisphere, but hers was dangerously low. We started her on supplements immediately and saw a drastic change in just weeks. I never imagined that one little vitamin could make such a change to a person. Her entire outlook on life was brighter; she was less exhausted and more focused. When Zandra was born, the doctors and nurses pressed me about the importance of giving vitamin D to infants. Although I trusted that it could be important, I also didn't have a lot of respect for those opinions, not if they were from the same school as the ones for flea bites in March. I was quite lax about giving supplements and now I wish I could go back in time and nourish her with vitamin D. I felt enormous guilt for having resisted, not because of my own intuition and investigation, but because I was angry with doctors. I was just glad that we were aware of the importance before any permanent damage was done.

The months that followed seemed to provide hope and promise to our fragile family. We were beginning to fall into a new normal with our new baby, and even with the visits the kids had with Kelley. For so long I felt I couldn't trust Kelley with the kids. I didn't feel they were safe when in his care. I heard stories of ATV crashes, bucking horses and capsizing canoes during their time with him that scared me to my core. I was hearing less of these stories, or perhaps I was just willing to let things go. I wanted so badly for the kids to have both of their parents and both of their stepparents working to support them. I adopted a view that the more love the merrier, and in Kelley's case, his common-law partner Carmen—a short, blond girl with some roundness that accounted for her motherly desire to keep goodies in full stock—was someone who looked after their dad well.

Time, as I found out, could either drag on the baggage of the past or heal it if I allowed my heart to open enough to see truths. I was learning to experience my feelings without judgment. I wasn't perfect, but I could feel and see that I was better than before. I was beginning to really like myself, and I now saw myself from an entirely different perspective than I ever had before. Life was by no means perfect, but I was feeling happy with where I was going, even if I knew I had a long way to go until I was who I truly desired to be.

I no longer wanted to become someone who looked good from my own perspective, but someone who *was* good. I was on a quest to find out exactly what God had created me for. Every day I tried to balance my own desires with the opportunities that crossed my way, dissecting each decision as to whether it allowed me to progress down my intended road or distracted me. Walking this path was excruciatingly slow in the beginning as I tried to use my intuition. It was like learning to read—every letter had a sound and grammar rules changed just when I thought I was understanding them. It took a while to learn to understand myself, what emotions and feelings were my own, contrasted with other people's, and again with messages from my own intuition.

I wanted to make some waves in this world, go out and shout about how my heart was changing. My life as a mother of four was exhausting and filled every waking hour. In the end, I reconciled that an authentic and present mother was exactly what God wanted me to be. Whatever else I needed to be would have to come in time, after sleep and caring for young kids.

Becoming this new me was scary, yet I felt brave. I became more open to opportunity and embraced the idea that I needed to become okay with challenging my fears. Growing up, Karen, Mom and Michael showed exceptional artistic talent. They were naturals at seeing the world through their pen or brush. They had an ability to accept both failure and success in their art and were praised for it. Karen decided to follow her talents, which led her to a career in graphic design. She could create art in any medium and was gifted in creating professional logos and media presentations, something our family of entrepreneurs has used to our advantage over the years.

I always admired her ability to create something beautiful and felt that I was artistic as well, although in different ways. Laura was equally talented with design and often used her creativity to make some of the most beautiful cakes for weddings and special occasions. I was always able to use my imagination in spaces, using colour, shapes and textures to create balance. I never took art classes in school, as I couldn't ever stand up to the personal rejection that my art wasn't as good as Karen's, so I never tried. It wasn't until I spent time with Vicky, the wife of one of Gord's coworkers, that I ever picked up a brush for the purpose of creating art. In time, I learned to accept my own creative style and have framed some acrylic paintings that I am proud of. I know my paintings are far from skilled, but I enjoy them just the same. I like to think that long after I'm gone, someone will have my painting on their wall and will get as much enjoyment from it as I do.

CHAPTER 6

Diabetes at School

GRADE 7 WAS SET TO begin just two weeks after Zandra's diagnosis. This meant a whole new school with new teachers and new routines. What once felt like an exciting time to see my firstborn enter a new phase now seemed scary, as I didn't know any of the teachers or administration. We were equipped for emergency low blood sugars, having been shown by the staff at the hospital how to use the emergency glucagon injection that releases stored sugar from the liver to the bloodstream if Zandra lost consciousness and couldn't be revived. We had her snacks and lunch pre-measured and her insulin pen ready for a lunch injection. I had gone in ahead of the first bell on the first day of school to talk to the administration. I wanted them to update their records of her condition and keep an eye out for her as she passed through the halls. Although first day was likely nothing but chaos for the school secretaries, they showed me nothing less than motherly attentiveness and assurance that I could call any time to get an update or be put through to her. I was far from ready to send Zandra to school, but, ready or not, we did it.

The diabetes diagnosis was challenging in ways I couldn't imagine. Zandra had wonderful, supportive friends who loved and cared for her, but their care had Zandra feeling the fear that they no doubt felt. Zandra noticed that things just weren't the same. In the days before school she went to her best friend's house to jump on the trampoline. She noticed that her friend was nervous about the activity and wanted her to stop jumping. When Zandra returned home, she was angry and hurt that her friend reacted the way she had. She explained, "They treat me like I'm a china doll! They're scared to play with me; they think that I'll pass out. I'm going to join hockey to show them that I'm just the same as they are." Most of Zandra's friends had played girls' hockey for several years, something that never interested Zandra until she had a point to prove. She was determined to prove to the world that diabetes didn't take away her strength, it gave her more.

Not only did Zandra have us sign her up for the hockey league even though she could barely skate, she was determined to join hockey academy with her school as well. The hockey academy had never accepted someone who hadn't played before, but they were willing to make an exception if she was committed to working hard. And hard it was. On the few occasions I watched the practices, I saw how far Zandra was behind all of the other players. I could see how skinny she was, as with undiagnosed diabetes she had been unable to build much muscle. I could see from the stands that Zandra not only had a physical setback, but she had to gain skill in the game, something that required mental endurance, the kind that comes from a fire within, the kind I knew she had but had yet to discover.

Hockey proved to be a blessing and a curse. Zandra's skill and endurance increased visibly every week. She worked exceptionally hard and earned a place as a worthy player in her league, but managing diabetes during the game, so early on in our journey, was very difficult. We learned that when she was on the ice, during practice and especially a game, the adrenalin blocked the insulin and she would often test high. In class we were taught to "feed for activity." There were guidelines about endurance and length of sport to indicate how much a diabetic person should consume to maintain a good blood sugar level throughout the activity. Zandra would consume sugar and see it increase her blood sugars into dangerous numbers, only for it to plummet into dangerously low levels in the short time it took to take off her gear and shower. Diabetes for her was unpredictable and random.

Often after games on the road, our team and the parents would go to a local restaurant to feed the hungry athletes. When a large team invades a small dining room like a small-town Boston Pizza without warning, it is often a long wait before the meals arrive. I wanted desperately for Zandra to feel normal and sit with her friends without having to deal with her disease. Very few teammates even knew of her diabetes and that's how she wanted it. She refused to do injections in front of anyone. She wouldn't even use her tester in their presence. I would wait for her to sneak off to a bathroom, silently trailing behind her to ask about her numbers in private, and was always greeted with a frustrated reply.

Insulin needs to be carefully calculated, and going to restaurants makes it really hard when you don't know how much food you're getting, or what you're hungry for. You can always add insulin, but if you've injected for a full meal and decide you're not actually that hungry, not eating is not an option. Insulin needs to be timed before a meal. Ideally, the injection should be fifteen minutes prior to eating so the insulin has a chance to work. Not doing so causes a high blood sugar spike, followed by a low. Different insulins peak at different times, and as she was on two different kinds, she had to be aware of when each one peaked. When a meal arrived late, which I had seen on more than one occasion, Zandra would be low and needing juice. When it arrived early, she had to wait the fifteen minutes while it went cold. Both scenarios were observed by her peers and made her extremely uncomfortable and visibly distressed.

One day before a practice I had a conversation with Marnie, her team manager. Marnie was a nurse and the mother of her friend and teammate, who coincidentally grew up with her dad as a type 1 diabetic. She was another godsend in my life. I always knew that when Zandra would sleep over at Marnie's house, she was in good, experienced hands. Marnie and I were both concerned that she was going to run into trouble hiding her condition, and that she was losing out on having her friends support her. I went in the locker room without telling Zandra beforehand and talked to the team about her diabetes. I spoke about what it meant to her game and what things she had to do outside of the ordinary to be safe, all the while deflecting the visual daggers coming my way from Zandra. After I said my piece and left, Marnie added to the team conversation by saying how teams are special and support one another. I knew I would experience the wrath of my very angry daughter, but I felt with everything in me it was the right move. I cried the entire drive home. I sobbed grief for not only myself, but also my daughter who had no control of the things going on around her. When she hurt, I hurt. That has been my honour and my burden since I first gave birth.

It took several weeks for Zandra's anger from feeling betrayed in front of her teammates to dissipate. I did my best in the following days to let her know that, above all, her health and survival were paramount for me and that being her mom didn't come with a simple playbook as hockey did. I apologized for hurting her and tried to open up a dialogue to learn how to handle future situations. No dialogue followed, but I prayed that she at the very least knew that I cared.

Grade 7 is a funny time. Anyone who has teenagers can probably relate to the absurdity of everyday junior-high life. Just six months prior in Grade 6, kids sat around lunch tables together, eating and playing games, then *bam!* Junior high comes and they don't want to eat in front of each other or talk about the same old activities. They worry about makeup and clothes—the big-box-store brands, which were once an easy go-to, were no longer an option; they were now an embarrassment. Girls would come out of school with what I called tarantula eyes: their eye makeup so thick it looked like they were peeking out of thick-legged spiders! My sweet daughter had become one of them.

I began to notice lunches coming home and a lot of snacking outside of meals. Blood sugars weren't being recorded for our next checkup, nor were food ratios jotted down. These things mattered, but not to a teenager. During several check-ins, her doctor and nurses urged her to keep her records or at least make a consistent plan, but I could tell that their recommendations were falling on deaf ears. The more I tried to involve myself, the greater the friction grew between us. Every time we went to the clinic, the nurses took a test that measures the average blood sugars for the previous three months, known as an A1C. Zandra's were dangerously low for a person her age. This indicated that she was having lows a lot more frequently than we knew. I received a stressed call once from her endocrinologist explaining that it was a matter of when, not if, Zandra would suffer serious consequences from low blood sugar. I fully understood the doctor but felt there was little I could do to get through to my independent daughter, as she had that giant chip on her shoulder. I knew that what appeared to be anger on the outside projected the fear from within. All I could do was walk a delicate line of monitoring her from a distance and pray that God would keep her safe.

During her Grade-7 year, her treatment team at the Stollery Children's Hospital recommended she consider getting an insulin pump. They were about to start a new round of pump-therapy classes and encouraged her to join. We were cautioned that a pump likely wouldn't change Zandra's A1C, but it could make life easier on a daily basis, as it eliminated the need to inject with every meal. It afforded freedom, allowing her to snack, eat light meals and even skip meals if she chose. The insulin pump is the most advanced tool for mimicking a natural pancreas. It uses only fast-acting insulin that is delivered in micro-dose spurts through the bloodstream. There were several downsides, however. The pump is connected to a person through an infusion site. This is a small tube that is placed under the skin, where it remains, which is uncomfortable to wear and must be moved to a new location every couple of days. There may be problems with making sure the pump site is connected properly and changed regularly, and it still requires the user to calculate every bite. The pump came at a cost of roughly seven thousand dollars and wasn't covered by either of our insurance plans. At this time, the Alberta government didn't recognize diabetes as a disability and didn't fund the pump. It seemed crazy to me that our government didn't recognize the very disease that was disabling my daughter's teenage life. There happened to be a lot of push from professionals and affected people who were advocating for a change. I made sure that my name made it to the list that helped sway the government's opinion just a few years later.

Zandra was able to try a loaner pump for a trial period, using saline rather than insulin, so we could see how it felt without the burden of having to understand how it worked. We had heard from every person in our social group who had one that it was the best thing to happen since they had been diagnosed. There wasn't a single bad review. The nurses set her up and showed her the basics. Most wearers of the pump found that attaching the infusion site to the stomach worked best, so we tried it first. It was a very painful experience for her, as she felt every move. It turned out that she didn't have enough of a fat layer on her stomach and the infusion was very uncomfortable on the muscle. We tried to change spots: arms, hips, leg—all had a similar problem. Zandra was still too lean to wear the pump comfortably, but we gave it a go anyhow.

That evening, Zandra tried to find a place where the pump was inconspicuous. The worst thing in her teenage mind would be for someone to notice it. She tried what the diabetic nurse did with hers, placing it between her cleavage, but she didn't have much of a cushion to work with. She almost always wore yoga pants without pockets, so we tried placing it in a hoodie pocket. The clear infusion line was visible from under her shirt to her pocket. We tried a fanny pack, but that was way too uncool and out of the question. During the night, she tried to keep it tucked into her pyjamas, but it kept pulling and was very uncomfortable. By the morning, she was an even more ornery teen than usual.

During the first class, her math teacher, the one who was also diabetic, just happened to be going through adult pump-therapy classes for his own pump. He had been a diabetic and was diagnosed around the same age as Zandra. As a runner and overall healthy person, he maintained a healthy balance and was a great example to all his students. He noticed Zandra's pump from her pocket, along with the infusion line, and discretely asked about it. He was excited that they could support each other. By the end of math class, Zandra had pulled off her pump completely. Although her teacher was discrete, she was mortified that he was able to notice it. That was it. Less than twenty-four hours after the trial started, it came to screeching halt.

As summer approached, the uneasiness began to creep in. Ordinarily we would send Zandra off to ranch camp for a week or two. She had attended Circle Square Ranch for several years, a camp in southern Alberta in an area by Halkirk. This camp has over 320 acres overlooking Paintearth Coulee. This Christian camp, with plenty of outdoor activities and horses, was always a highlight for her. She looked forward to bunking with her friends and devouring the camp food. I wanted to give her the same summer experiences that she loved, but was fearful that she wouldn't be able to manage her blood sugars. I knew she wouldn't want anyone else to know about her disease, and I was certain she wouldn't ask for help if she needed it. The nurses at the Stollery offered a diabetes-friendly option. They suggested a camp referred as D Camp, otherwise known as Camp Jean Nelson. This camp was located in the foothills of the picturesque Rocky Mountains of Alberta. Campers sleep in dorms with groups similar in age. The part that quelled my fears was that there were three camp counsellors per cabin, hired by Diabetes Canada, many of whom were type 1 diabetics themselves. They offered twenty-four-hour supervision and oversaw each camper's blood sugars. It was even rumoured that Paul Brandt had worked at the camp as a nurse before he became a country music star, while he worked at the Calgary Children's Hospital.

Zandra was always adventurous, so it didn't surprise me that she agreed to this new camp, although she was sad not to return to her familiar camp with her old friends. She seemed skeptical about taking part in an activity-based camp with other diabetic kids, with camp leaders looking after them as if they were infants.

We decided to drive to the town of Bragg Creek together and spend a few days hiking and staying in a log cabin bed and breakfast before I dropped her off at the nearby camp for the week. We had no plans for our days, just two girls out for an adventure to get into a great frame of mind. This was the first time we had ever gone away with just the two of us for a trip and I was excited. We stopped off in Red Deer for some scrapbooking supplies—we had some photos of our trip to Disneyland that we planned to memorialize if we were bored. We packed up our minivan—affectionately known as Miles—and were soon captivated by the Rocky Mountain views, something that never gets old for either of us. We immediately loved the cabin in the woods and our hosts were genuinely gracious and hospitable. We rented a room in the loft of an A-frame that provided a beautiful scenic view of the mountains.

Rain seemed to drizzle continually, but we were ready with raincoats and umbrellas. We hiked through the rain, walked through the small but beautiful art gallery and drove along the quiet back roads. On our second day, we came across a group of wild horses, something that neither one of us realized would be there. We stopped the van and watched in awe as the group—tentatively at first—warmed up to us and came close with their foals. There was something transformative in my soul being that close to those horses. I knew Zandra felt the same way. From that point on, we realized that we had shared an unspoken miracle. Zandra had long loved riding horses and was taking regular lessons. She always insisted that horses regulated her blood sugars, and somehow she was right, they often did. Once we even charted out her riding days and correlated them with her better days.

Our trip was a much-needed respite for me as well. Just months prior, I was diagnosed with thyroid disease. My symptoms came on slowly and were hard to recognize. I had been living somewhat functionally while raising a young family, not to mention managing Zandra's diabetes, and I hadn't realized that I wasn't well myself. I felt utterly exhausted and was too tired to notice my hair loss, including the loss of most of my eyebrows. It wasn't until I was carpooling with our friends to a soccer game that I understood just how out of sorts I was. Two of the mothers on the team were in the vehicle with me when I started nodding off in the back seat. They were concerned about my constant exhaustion and demanded that I get my thyroid tested, as both of them suffered from a thyroid condition themselves. My friend Cindy noticed my apathy toward my own health and warned me, "Thyroid disease goes far beyond feeling tired. It seeps into your entire body until you no longer care about the fact that you feel terrible." She was right. I didn't care about my condition and I needed to look after myself. I made sure to see a doctor and have my blood tested. Within days, I received a call to return to the doctor's office where I was told of my thyroid condition. After taking medications and committing to take care of myself, I was beginning to feel more like my old self and looked forward to spending time in the mountains with Zandra.

The camp was an overall positive experience, yet she only went for that one year. Zandra enjoyed the activities and the backup knowledge of the counsellors, but it was clear to her that her independence was gone. It wasn't the same as Circle Square Ranch. She missed riding the horses at camp as well as her old friends. As much as the camp tried to make testing blood sugars and overseeing insulin the lesser focus of the trip, the sheer amount of kids deemed that impossible in her eyes. All focus was on diabetes and less on adventure from her defiant perspective.

Low blood sugars continued to be a problem for Zandra. I was getting better at catching on and attributing her moods to her blood sugars. I began noticing that she would slow down as if she were drowsy and tired, and, conversely, the irritability that comes with the highs. On the weekends when the older kids went with Kelley, I insisted on being kept in the loop regarding blood sugars. This version of helicopter mom became a problem for both Kelley and Zandra, who didn't appreciate being reminded of the severity of unchecked diabetes. I was noticing several alarming numbers on Zandra's tester when I would review it after she returned from her weekends. I would send several emails and place several calls to Kelley about parental accountability, as well as to Zandra, explaining that if she wanted to be away she needed to be okay asking for help when needed.

During the summer of 2013, the kids went to be with their dad for the week. We resumed the familiar schedule of one week with dad alternating with a week with me throughout the summer, making exceptions for camps and activities the kids were involved in. Always ignoring my feelings of fear, I would send them off and do my best to connect once or twice a week to touch base. When they were away, I would take advantage of having less traffic around the house to get some home projects accomplished. During one of the weeks, I decided to finish painting the upstairs hallway, which was open to the family room on the main level and didn't match the colour I'd painted that room a couple of months prior. The weather was perfect to open the windows and let the house vent. As I was painting over the neutral beige, I had a feeling I should call to check on the kids. The feeling was nagging, so I decided to set down the soppy paint roller and make the call. Kelley answered his phone and assured me that the kids were all doing well. I inquired about Zandra's blood sugars, getting to the point of why I called in the first place. He told me the all too familiar story of how everything was in control in his house. This never sat well with me, because I knew that diabetes was imperfect at the best of times and Zandra's testers told a different story following other visits.

I insisted on being put in touch with Zandra but was told that she was napping. Napping for Zandra was unusual. Even as an infant, I struggled to get her to close her eyes for five minutes. She's just never been one to need much sleep, but what do I know? Maybe the extended summer days had caught up with her. I decided to let it go and get back to painting. After a while, the feeling hadn't gone. I still felt like I needed to get an update, at the very least. I decided to call back, risking being called out for meddling. I phoned again and was told by Kelley that Zandra couldn't come to the phone. I insisted on talking to Olivia or Joseph. Olivia suddenly came on the phone with a worried tone in her voice. I asked what had been going on and she indicated that she was worried for Zandra. She said that Zandra was hardly responding to her, and it was making her scared. I asked some questions about how long she had been sleeping and asked her to try to wake her with me on the phone. I could hear a weary voice struggling to speak on the other end. My adrenalin kicked in. I told her to hand the phone over to her dad.

When Kelley got back on the phone I asked him to try to rouse her. He couldn't. I asked him to call 911, but he didn't think that was necessary. I was still in shock, wondering if I had it wrong. Maybe she really was just exhausted and sleepy. Maybe I was making something out of nothing. At the same time, I was angry. I told Kelley to give her as much juice as he could and asked him to meet me with her on the highway. The plan was for us both to leave and meet at a halfway point. I fought the entire drive with my decision to drive to her or whether I should have insisted on calling 911. When I met up with Kelley's truck, I was struck that Zandra couldn't walk. Kelley carried her to my vehicle. I was a tornado of emotion, whirling with anger, concern and dread. When Kelley brought her to my passenger seat she was barely conscious. I wasn't prepared for what I saw, but I had juice boxes with me and immediately started pouring juice into her mouth, watching her slowly sip it while much of it ended up spilling back out. I struggled, yet managed to get the majority of the box down her while driving to the nearest hospital. I called the emergency on-call number for the diabetes clinic and left a message. Someone called me back right away, within minutes. I explained what was happening and was assured that the fact Zandra was somewhat conscious was a good sign. I was instructed to continue providing juice, and to take her blood sugars once I was able to. I have no recollection of whom I spoke with on the phone, but their calm manner helped me get through the moment and make decisions that I needed to make.

As I was nearing Camrose, I decided that I would take Zandra home rather than continue to the hospital. She was conscious, although she still couldn't speak. I knew that if I needed to get her there, the hospital was five minutes from my house. When I got home, Zandra was at least able to walk, although she needed assistance. I took her upstairs to lie in my bed and tested her blood sugar. She was still low, so I continued to feed her juice until her blood sugars returned to normal. I logged everything in detail, down to the times and actions taken. I've done this since the kids were babies. I never wanted to rely on a parent's exhausted memory of when medications were administered for fevers. I call it their "charts," just like in a hospital. For Zandra, these charts would be emailed to the diabetes clinic for help so that I had support to get her well.

Once Zandra's blood sugars were out of the danger zone, it took her many hours until she could stand on her feet properly and even talk. I laid in bed with her for the next couple of nights, feeling her breath against mine, just like she was a newborn again. When she regained her ability to talk, she told me that she thought she was dying. She said she felt confident that her time had come to an end. My heart broke because I knew she had been close. I knew that her time would have come to an end if I hadn't listened to my inner voice. Thinking about what almost happened has been a driving force for wanting to share the seriousness of this disease with the world. The worst almost happened to us. It can and has happened to others.

After experiencing such a potentially fatal situation, I needed to know what went wrong. It was a simple mistake: Zandra had low blood sugar going into lunch. She wanted to take her insulin and eat but forgot an important step: *Never take insulin when blood sugars are low.* When blood sugars are low and insulin is given, it will only lower it further, possibly creating a life or death situation. Further, when experiencing low blood sugars, vision and concentration are blurred, making mistakes in dosage more likely. Zandra felt that this might have been what happened to her. She realized after the fact that it was hard to see the numbers on her insulin pen, and she likely overdosed.

Mistakes can and do happen, so taking the initiative to notice behaviours, ask questions and follow up with checking was vital.

Nobody wants to be the unpopular parent, but for a diabetic child it becomes paramount to make sure that their actions are overseen by an adult, even though they may resist.

The toll of this experience was both physical and emotional. The physical adjustment was long and difficult. Soon after her blood sugars levelled out, they began to climb. This is something that as a parent I've seen time and time again. After a severe low, high blood sugar often follows. Zandra's body was flooded with sugar to get her functioning, but when her body caught up and had too much, the highs came. This part was difficult. Her body felt weak and sick and we were both scared to administer insulin. Although the clinic had always been helpful, it's down to each individual to learn how to adjust for themselves. We decided for Zandra that she would take small doses of insulin, drink lots of water and walk, although her pace was slow for the first days. This severe low has been to date the worst I have ever seen for her. I know full well that there are parents who have experienced much worse, their children going into seizures which required them to administer glucagon injections. My heart breaks for what they've had to witness and manage. After this experience, Zandra's body completely refused to perceive low blood sugars again. It's as if her body lost its ability to send the signal of distress. This consequence, called *hypoglycemic unawareness*, continues to put her at risk to this day.

Intellectually, Zandra understood that her disease could take her life. She realized that, although she was good at managing her own blood sugars and administering insulin, sometimes she needed help. She had what I hoped was a healthy dose of fear, enough to take her needs seriously but not too much to clip her wings and prevent her from reaching her potential. I hoped at the time that she understood my role and sympathized with me. I wanted her to know and understand that I didn't want to set out limits and check in on her because I didn't trust her, but that I needed to make sure she was safe. But that wasn't the case yet. Teenagers can't see around corners. They tend to see from their own perspective, building first their own ideas until their brain is fully developed. Until then, they tend to lack perspective. She wouldn't understand other perspectives until she fully understood her own. So when I limited her time with her dad for her own safety, she didn't understand, she only knew how it made her feel. She was angry with me and made sure I knew it.

I was terrified that what happened could happen again. I needed assurance that the same scenario wouldn't play out again before she went back, so I asked Kelley to retake the training at the Stollery, or to take any steps that demonstrated that he understood how to help next time. Legally I had to comply with the terms of our divorce agreement, so that meant sending the kids to him for a couple of weekends a month, but I was willing to challenge that in this case and hold Zandra back. I didn't have an idea how long it would take for my request to be fulfilled, I just needed to hear that there was some ownership of responsibility about what happened. I needed to hear remorse for trying to cover up a situation that almost turned fatal. I wanted to open up the lines of communication so that if the same situation or one similar happened again, I could trust him to put his own feelings aside and call me, or access emergency help for himself. I understood that Zandra was angry with me, but I prayed that at the very least she could trust that I would keep her safe.

Months soon passed and we were looking into the holiday season. Typically we shared the holidays, with me bringing the kids over to Kelley's house on Christmas Day and picking them up on New Year's Eve. This year would be different. I wouldn't be able to go that long trusting the life of my child to anyone, even another parent, who didn't understand diabetes. In the end, we compromised on staying over two nights with promised check-ins after every blood test, even though Kelley took no steps toward learning from the Stollery. If I couldn't trust Kelley to be responsible, I needed to trust Zandra. She was clearly affected by my decision and her frustration at me was understandable. We needed to start somewhere, so I decided to work with her. She didn't like my oversight of her blood sugars, but she seemed to understand my compromise, thank God. I also tried to empower Olivia and Joseph to see the signs of distress and encouraged them to call for help. I let them know that nobody would ever be angry if it turned out not to be an emergency, as this could save her life one day.

We continued with short trips with frequent communication that I oversaw through to the summer. Luckily, shorter trips were quite acceptable to a teenage girl who didn't want to be away from her friends for too long. I didn't have to be the bad guy much longer. She only ever wanted to be away a day or two on her own terms. By the following year, trust had indeed been built. I could trust that when Zandra felt she didn't know what to do, or how to treat her highs or lows, she would ask for my help. If I didn't know the answers, we would seek them together. Before long, she would be calling and emailing the clinic herself with questions and participated much more fully in her appointments.

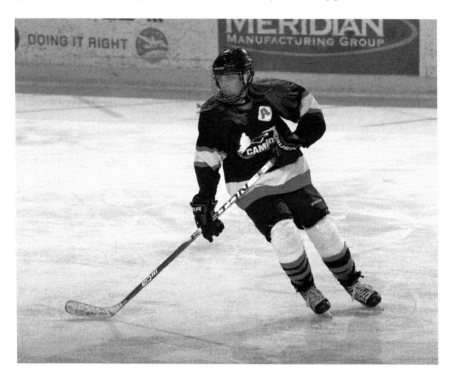

Game night

CHAPTER 7

Iceland

DIABETES WAS A SHOCK TO my system. I never asked for it to be a part of my life, nor Zandra's. The weight of diagnosis and the steep learning curve to simply manage our day-to-day lives took a toll. They say that people with diabetes are twice as likely to suffer from depression and anxiety-related conditions. I have no doubt that the sheer number of sacrifices that need to be made in order to live with diabetes can significantly alter the mental health of those who are diagnosed. I also know, as a parent of a diabetic, that the stress has altered my own mental health at times as well. I got to a point where the burden became increasingly hard to bear. I recalled researching diabetes the night of diagnosis, as I was desperately trying to assure Zandra that she would continue to live a normal life. At that time, Zandra and I had homed in on Iceland as a destination for running events that raised awareness of diabetes, and I now decided to dive deeper into something positive.

The website for Diabetes Canada indicated that the signup for the upcoming Iceland run was open. I mentioned this to Zandra and her interest was piqued. As an equestrian rider, she was familiar with the Icelandic horse and was immediately taken with that destination. She knew that none of her friends had gone there and that it would be an adventure.

After signing up, we were quickly assigned support people—not only for our run, but to help us meet our fundraising goals of over six thousand dollars each. I had been running in half marathons for a couple of years and had a good idea what to expect from the race, but I had never been involved with a team run. I planned to do another half marathon, which is around twenty kilometres, but the rules stated that as Zandra was fourteen years old, she could only run the 10K. I decided to run the 10K with her so I could keep my eye on her performance, in case she needed any care before the finish line. I knew that Zandra would be reluctant to carry her own sugar or tester, so, anticipating this, I needed to keep pace and have these things on me just in case.

To kick off our fundraising, Gord, who was still a Crown prosecutor at that time, had some really good connections. He wrote a letter outlining Zandra's condition and asked his colleagues for support, which came flooding in with letters describing how each one had been affected by a loved one's struggle with diabetes. The feeling of connectedness with all our supporters cultivated a love and respect that I hadn't previously drawn upon, and the upcoming trip took on a whole new meaning for me. I had set out on this journey to expand Zandra's horizon. After watching her bravely face so many obstacles in her life, including hypoglycemic unawareness, I felt it was time to grow our understanding, support vital work in diabetes and experience a new part of the world. By participating in the fundraising, I was humbled by the combined effort with people from around the world. The excitement and enthusiasm of having so many engaged participants created a powerful experience for us both.

Although the initial support allowed us to meet our first fundraising goal, we still had a long way to go. We decided we needed an event. At the time of planning, the girls were playing soccer. I spent a lot of time on the sidelines with other moms, talking about our children's lives and sharing our plans to go to Iceland. One of the parents, Marie, immediately volunteered to help with organizing a fundraising evening with a silent auction. Marie had experience doing events and was well-connected with the community to seek out donations. To drum up the attendance, the local paper published our story along with a photo on the front page. The exposure from this article not only drew in a large crowd for the evening of the event, but also connected us with many other people who also lived with diabetes.

The community of Camrose overwhelmed me with its generous donations and support. People who hardly knew us were handing over cash donations to assist with our mission. With all of the donations, we had more than enough funds to meet our financial obligation. The unexpected upside from the fundraising we did was the platform it gave Zandra to speak. For so long, she had tried to hide her diabetes, feeling shame from it and fearing rejection. Through the experience, like it or not, her secret was exposed.

The trip to Iceland finally came to fruition in August of 2014. The day before we were set to leave, news of an impending volcanic eruption threatened our trip. In 2010, a large volcano in Iceland released approximately 150,000 tons of CO_2 each day, causing a massive ash cloud in European skies that affected air travel throughout the continent. Seismic activity showed that another volcano was picking up and fountains of lava began spilling from an old fissure. If this volcano erupted, there was no telling what impact it would have on our run, much less our ability to return home. The threat of a volcanic eruption secretly added to the thrill and excitement of the trip.

Diabetes Canada immediately addressed the situation and gave their go-ahead. The next day we were headed as scheduled to Iceland! The flight was the longest I had been on, at six hours direct from Edmonton. Iceland Air felt quite deluxe compared to the economy carriers that we were both accustomed to, offering proper meals and delicious foreign snacks. The trip felt surreal. As we began our descent, we could clearly see the giant formations of icebergs in the water and how much of them rest below the surface of the water, revealing only the literal "tip of the iceberg." We were able to observe these astounding features of the coastal community while watching Greenland come into focus.

We arrived at the airport early in the morning. It was in the town of Keflavík, about thirty minutes' drive from where we were staying in Reykjavík. We planned to take a shuttle to our hotel once we cleared customs and picked up our baggage. The airport was unfamiliar and rather different from ones I'd been through before. I was surprised when we were stopped at security directly after the flight. My other travel experiences allowed me to leave once our baggage was claimed.

After landing on the airstrip, I noticed Zandra was quiet. I asked her about her blood sugars and she ignored my question. I decided to accept that her mood and behaviour were likely a result of a long overnight flight, and understand that if I was being watched I would likely be just as slow. The weight of responsibility travelling with Zandra and her needs was always palpable, but I decided to look past it. As we were lining up in the airport, we were directed to grab bins and place all of our carry-on items in them. As we were shuffling through the scanners, it became clear to me that Zandra's blood sugars were low. She was moving even more slowly and wasn't responding as she should. As she was hypoglycemic unaware, she likely didn't even know herself that her blood sugars were dropping.

Prior to leaving on our trip, I packed some dried fruit bars in my suitcase, something that worked perfectly for low blood sugars. Zandra had been working hard to clean up her diet, avoiding artificial sugars and preservatives, and these snacks fit her criteria. Zandra's favourite and most effective treatment, however, has always been drinking juice; she's found that juice raises her blood sugar faster than any other sugar. We made sure that we bought a large juice after we cleared customs in Edmonton to have on hand for our flight. We knew that there was plenty of juice on the aircraft should we need some as well.

Our bags were held up with the attendant who was doing the scanning. There were two problems: the cooling pack, which we use in her insulin bag, and her unopened juice. As the airport staff was convening to discuss the unknown cooling gel in the pack, Zandra began to hold the conveyer for support. I asked the staff to hand us the juice and they explained that they couldn't hand over any liquids. I drew their attention to the unopened seal and let them know that we purchased the juice after clearing security in Edmonton. I explained to them why we needed it immediately and pointed to Zandra, who by now couldn't even focus on the discussion. They were clearly unaware of what diabetes was and didn't understand the magnitude of the situation. My pledge to raise awareness for diabetes had already begun. As the discussion grew into more of an argument, with a growing and exhausted crowd behind us, I realized I wasn't going to win. Inside I was scolding myself as the responsible adult for not carrying another form of sugar—if only

I had packed a Fruit to Go in my purse as well as my checked luggage. A young lady who worked with Iceland Air noticed Zandra, as she was growing more lethargic by the minute. She suggested that I take Zandra to a vending machine in another part of the airport to purchase a new juice. This was going to be my best option.

Before we left for our trip, I looked into getting Icelandic currency, called *króna*. The bank in Camrose had to order it and it would take several days. I had asked other people who had visited Iceland if they thought I should leave with the converted currency and they all assured me that it was easy to head to a bank while there, or even use my credit card for all purchases. Some of my friends hadn't even bothered to obtain króna, they always used their credit cards. Now, standing in the airport, I was fearful that my decision was a mistake. I had no idea if the vending machines would work with Canadian funds. As we left the security area and set out to find the vending machine, the same attendant took it upon herself to escort us there. She let me know that the machines took other currency and was willing to purchase the juice for us if we didn't have any. She helped by grabbing Zandra's carry-on and offered to help with her other arm when Zandra could hardly walk. Once we reached the machine, I had my wallet ready and plunked in my coins, not caring if a soft drink was our only option. There was an apple juice clearly visible, so I selected it without second thought. I quickly popped the top and gave it to Zandra—she had already found a place on the floor to sit, as she could no longer stand steady on her feet.

The airline worker was very apologetic and said that she would be letting her coworkers know what happened so it wouldn't happen again. I made myself a promise to always carry Fruit to Go with me from that point forward. As much as Zandra wanted to be independent, she still needed me. I could clearly recall myself at her age and my fight for autonomy. I felt like I was between both worlds, understanding both sides with clarity. I felt as though a download of information was given to me, like a computer backup. I had an upgrade that allowed my own ego to step aside and let her have her space. I knew the way forward was to stay close enough to support her when she needed me, and in the meanwhile accept the feelings of rejection from those same boundaries. I reframed my own feelings in an instant.

When we boarded the shuttle to the airport, we met a couple of ladies from Edmonton who were part of the same run. One of them also had diabetes and the other was her friend who was there to support her. She appeared to be enjoying the carefree days of her youth. As she spoke, I could hear my mom's voice chime in: "'Tis better to be silent and thought a fool, than to speak and remove all doubt." I enjoyed this silent musing and we headed toward Reykjavík. We parted ways with our new friends once we reached the hotel. While we were waiting in the lineup to leave our bags at the desk, Zandra leaned in to tell me something she obviously wanted to keep quiet while in the company of the ladies we had met. She informed me that she knew how this beautiful young mother stayed so slender. While on the shuttle, Zandra asked her about her blood sugar control. She was giggly and evasive, replying, "I'm often running too high, but that's okay with me, although it's not healthy." As soon as she said it I knew exactly what she meant, although I had no idea that my daughter did as well.

I was warned early on in our diabetes journey that there is an eating disorder specific to diabetics, coined as "diabulimia." The diabetic uses insulin manipulation to keep their blood sugars running higher, to the point where they create ketones as a source of energy, which can lead to weight loss. This type of eating disorder is extremely dangerous and one that I never wanted Zandra to know of. But here she was, telling me all about it. She told me that she realized for herself that when her blood sugars ran high, she noticed weight loss and figured it out. Not only did she know of it, she was able to see it in others. Thankfully, it seemed that she was condemning this foolish behaviour.

When we arrived at the hotel in downtown Reykjavík, we fell in love. The hotel was a transformed paint factory and close to the water. The décor throughout the lobby felt like walking through the showrooms of a Swedish furniture store and we couldn't wait to see our room. The problem was, it was just after eight in the morning and we didn't have access to our room until the afternoon. There was a growing number of those of us arriving for the diabetes run in the same situation. Standing around, we had an opportunity to informally meet one another, including the organizers and coaches.

We had several hours before we had access to our much-needed beds, so we decided to head out and find a place with nice coffee and something to eat. Before we left, I opened our luggage and grabbed a few packages of the Fruit to Go's. I wasn't going to be caught again without emergency sugar on hand. We both enjoyed exploring while walking through the historic downtown, seeing the bright coastal colours of the painted buildings. It looked exactly like the photos in the magazines! We found a quaint café and decided to settle in for breakfast. Before we ordered, I wanted to be sure my credit card would be accepted, knowing that I didn't have any króna. The server indicated that they were happy to accept all cards and payment types, which was a relief for me. We each ordered lattes, which to our surprise came with beautiful leaf designs poured into the foam. We also ordered a light breakfast that would suffice until our next meal. We decided to sit down awhile and enjoy the atmosphere while eating and come up with a plan of what we'd like to do next. While Zandra was finishing her last bites and taking a quick restroom break, I went up to the counter to pay. Apparently, during our breakfast, the café had their banking system rehauled and they were unable get credit cards to work. The server was very apologetic and tried to explain where the bank was as best as he could in English. Not taking out cash ahead of time had turned out to be a mistake.

I decided to leave Zandra with the last sips of her latte while I quickly headed out to find the bank. I didn't want the staff to think I would ditch the bill, although they were more concerned about getting their system back in order than my leaving. Lacking a keen sense of direction, I ventured out, being sure to recall landmarks to find my way back. As I made my way through downtown streets, I came upon a stately-looking building with giant columns and prominent features. I found myself grateful that banks are often built with a measure of extravagance, and this one was fairly easy to spot. I headed into the large building and was grateful for signage that was translated in English. The transaction itself was easy and I pulled out enough króna to get me through the days that we would be there, should we need cash again. After the bank, I recalled my steps back to the coffee shop like Hansel and Gretel, deliberately recalling markers to find my way.

After settling the bill for breakfast, we strolled through the streets of downtown Reykjavík. We meandered into the residential neighbourhoods, following our curiosity and sense of adventure. While enjoying the architecture of the neighbourhood homes, we noticed that many of them, along with their landscaping, were similar to ours in Alberta. We identified several plants that we had in our own garden, ones that I didn't know the names of and some that I did. We stopped to pet several trusting cats relaxing in sunbeams, stretched out on the concrete in front of their homes. These familiar surroundings in a new land made us feel right at home.

Travelling to Iceland gave us our first experience of adjusting insulin in a different time zone. We'd never worried about the one- to two-hour adjustments, but as this was a six-hour difference, we had to plan differently. The Stollery made that process easy. All they asked for were our travel times and they returned the email with an adjustment that made sense for the way there and back. Because Zandra was on injections, she used two different types of insulin. One was fast-acting, used to bring down the sugar in her meals, otherwise known as a "bolus" insulin. The other one was a long-acting insulin, taken at the same time each day, which provided a continual small dose at all times, known as a "basal" insulin. In a healthy, non-diabetic person, there is only one insulin, which is continuously being released throughout the body. Although the insulin is fairly consistent, it does have its peaks and must be adjusted for this type of travel. The Stollery ended up splitting the dose of her long-range insulin in half the first night to allow for the difference. After that, we would resume the usual amount. This worked quite well in the end, giving us confidence that travel is something that can be managed. While we explored through the streets of Reykjavík, I was comforted that the professionals had managed the guesswork and I was able to let go and enjoy some aspects of the trip.

I hadn't bothered to buy a power converter for my phone, as the hotel information indicated they offered them as complimentary to their guests. My cell phone was running low, and at the time we checked in the attendant had told us that all of their converters were loaned out. They suggested we check back early the next day, while guests were checking out and before new ones arrived. The following morning, however, the attendant informed me that they were still out and didn't know when they would have another one available. My phone was in the last ten percent of its charge, so I decided to set out and find a converter at a nearby store. Zandra and I went out walking to the nearest hardware store, which, according to Google Maps, ended up being several kilometres away. Ever since Zandra was about ten, she rarely walked with me; rather, she walked ahead of me, inferring that I was the slower one who should keep pace with her. She walked along quickly and stubbornly, knowing full well that I wasn't willing to keep up her pace. She almost always walked this way at home, but when we were out in a foreign place I didn't expect her to keep up the charade, but she was. I never knew if she walked ahead to prove a point or because she was embarrassed to be seen with me. I've always been a brisk walker—at a height of five foot eight with long legs I was taller than her, yet somehow slower. At one point along our walk to the store, Zandra had walked so far ahead of me it was hard to see her. All I could see was her frame with the swinging ponytail of her long brunette hair. I was frustrated. I decided to pretend as though I didn't care. It took a lot of effort, but the more I walked alone, the easier it became, until I almost didn't care.

The giant hardware store looked almost exactly like the ones back home, but with everything written in Icelandic. When we walked in, the layout was familiar, and it struck me how globalized hardware stores are. I quickly found our way to the bins full of power converters displayed in an orderly fashion. They were nicely labelled by country, so we easily found the one that read CANADA that would work for us without having to ask for assistance. We found the power converter much faster than I had expected to. I quickly did the conversion from króna to Canadian funds in my head and realized that the cost was quite reasonable as well. Once we paid for the converter, we walked back to the hotel the same way we arrived: me trailing several feet behind Zandra, acting as though I had come alone.

Sleeping has always been a challenge for me. I've never been a good sleeper, but as I had a diabetic child and had to check blood sugars through the night on top of being in an unfamiliar place, sleep was near impossible. I found myself awake night after night, reading in the bathroom as to not disturb Zandra, who was sleeping in the bed next to mine, or quietly watching TV with the volume turned low. I've learned to cope well on little sleep, but when it came to race day, I felt like I had already run a race before we started.

I had skipped the pre-race run with our group the day before, trying in vain for a nap that never came. The organizers had several planned events, including a couple of group meals where we could gather and talk about the work that was being done in the field of diabetes. The organizers highlighted the successes accomplished by our fundraising, and acknowledged Canada as a world leader in policy around diabetes as well as in research. I typically have never enjoyed these types of group rah-rah events, but this felt different. I genuinely felt that I was not only appreciated, but that I was part of something that served a need in the world. I was proud of myself for the effort, and to all those who supported us on our trip. It was truly a moment when words would not suffice to express the immensity of my gratitude. I was especially proud of Zandra, who had not asked for this disease but was willing to be a change-maker, and she wanted to ensure that nobody had to face the challenges that she's had to.

The hotel offered a continental breakfast unlike any I had ever had. The portions were small but provided a considerably generous selection. They had several types of eggs, breads, butters and jams, along with fruits, vegetables and an assortment of pickles. Every breakfast was a luxury that didn't go unnoticed. With the constant refreshing of our coffees and plates, I felt more like a queen than a race participant.

When race day arrived, I was astounded to see such large crowds drawing in. I had understood that there were many different organizations from around the world coming together in Reykjavík for the race, but I wasn't prepared for what I saw: there were thousands of runners! There were so many runners that each participant had to select a finishing time so they could be corralled at the start by that estimate. I've since learned this format wasn't new for large runs, but it was nothing like the runs I had participated in up to that point. Zandra immediately chose her time. She was faster than me, but it was important to me that we stay together, especially after the airport fiasco. I knew that I was exhausted and didn't want to push myself to finish inside an hour, but Zandra insisted that she would be forty-five minutes. I contemplated joining her, but was worried that I would occupy space that much faster runners needed. The decision needed to be made quickly, and in that moment I reluctantly agreed to let my fourteen-year-old daughter stand alone amongst thousands to run. I was holding her tester and the sugar that we had brought and asked her to take it from me. "I'm not taking my sugar. There's juice along the way," she said. Before I could insist that she take her tester, she disappeared into the crowd.

I walked back toward the section for the longer run times and placed myself in the corral that anticipated the length at an hour. I was holding in anger and frustration, but mostly fear. Not just the normal parental fear of thousands of strangers all around in a foreign country, but of how dangerous this situation could be. I consoled myself that I'd rather be behind her than in front, so that if she slowed down or stopped I would spot her. I needed to keep scanning the large crowd just in case my fears were confirmed. I moved out of my place to find one of our Diabetes Canada volunteers, Diane. I explained the situation to her and she promised that she would also look out for Zandra. Diane had been involved in the run in Iceland for many years and didn't have the same apprehensions that I did. Her outward calmness worked to quell my inner freak-out. I placed myself back into the swelling line and waited for the race to start.

We started with a loud bang that was barely audible to the crowd as far back as we were. I was all set, my mission clear in my head. I stood waiting sentinel for three songs to cycle before the line even budged. When I finally began to move along, I recognized the song "Happy" by Pharrell Williams blasting on the loudspeakers. I was finally able to creep ahead into a slow jog. The song was infectious. Before long, I was bouncing through the crowds enjoying the race and the magnificent scenery of the black volcanic rock set against the deep blue hues of the ocean. As I ran, I kept Zandra's tester clenched in my hand and an eye out for her team shirt. When we had received our race package with our shirts, I was taken aback by the loud, gaudy colours of them; I never liked standing out and these shirts did just that. In that moment, I made a complete one-eighty and was now thankful for the gaudy tops so I could spot Zandra amongst the others.

Along the run, supporters cheered on from the sidelines and neighbouring balconies, using pots and pans as noisemakers. I embraced the support and allowed myself to genuinely feel the moment. I told myself that for as long as I lived, I would recall the sights, smells, feel and love that these strangers offered. It was a beautiful gift that I allowed myself, and one that I look back on time and time again with great thanksgiving. I was so absorbed in the moment that I felt as if I was on a runner's high for the entire duration of the race. I didn't stop or slow down, or even want to. I completed the race in an hour, but it flew by like never before in any run.

When the finish line was drawing near, I could see the swell of supporters ready to high-five the finishers. I was excited to be amongst the people being cheered and felt personal satisfaction with my run. I knew that Zandra must have already passed through, as I didn't see her or pass her on my way. I was excited to hear about her experience and compare stories. She would have no doubt seen the supporters and taken notice of the same panoramic views as I had along the way.

Once I reached the end, reality stabbed me like a knife. I didn't see Zandra anywhere. I had expected she would remain alongside the finish line to welcome me across. I could feel panic getting the better of me, twisting in my chest and pounding against my ribs. I searched frantically across the crowd for a Diabetes Canada volunteer, looking for the same race tank that I had on. I commanded myself to come across calm, yet I'm sure that my fear betrayed me. I managed to locate one of our volunteers and they appeased me, telling me that Zandra had finished a while ago and shouldn't be far. I knew from experience that after an activity, when the adrenalin wore off, her blood sugars could plummet and she wouldn't even notice. I was calculating timelines and trying to anticipate her blood sugars. I knew she didn't have juice stands anymore or money on her to purchase any if she needed it. I had to find her immediately. I started walking around the crowds, growing more frantic by the step.

The race ended near the parliament buildings and I desperately began to scour all of the lawns in the surrounding area. After about fifteen long, uneasy minutes, I found her. She said she wasn't sure where to find me and had decided to hang out past the crowds. She didn't appear bothered by my anxiety, which struck an immediate nerve. I was angered that she hadn't waited or offered an apology, as she could see I was visibly distraught. I had to see past my emotions quickly and insist she test her blood. I was still concerned that she was low and needed the sugar I was holding. After testing, we found that Zandra's levels were remarkably good, reminding me that I could never know when my concern would be validated—not that I ever wanted it to be.

The post-race banquet was nothing short of spectacular. Held in a historic building, we got to see some of the beautiful architecture within Iceland's capital. I was able to fully realize the enormousness of the trip in that final celebration. The total fundraising contribution amounted to a significant donation in the end. The amount raised by a small group of Canadians inspired me to vow to participate again. Zandra and I both enjoyed the banquet, feeling proud of what we had accomplished and knowing that we helped to make a difference. Now that the race was over, we were able to look forward to the other activities that we had planned for our trip.

The evening of the race was Reykjavík's annual Culture Night. Tens of thousands of people went to the capital to celebrate with food, activities and live bands set up on enormous concert stages. After the banquet, we decided to walk through the streets and get a feel for the celebration. Most of the streets were closed off to traffic and allowed pedestrians to have the right of way. Shops opened their doors and placed sale items, samples and games outside. The vibe was exhilarating and fun. The entire city came to life and carried on through the night. We walked through the streets and stayed long enough to enjoy some of the open-air concert. The performers were singing in a foreign language, but that didn't take away from the experience. As the sun set, people began donning glow sticks around their necks and wrists. When the sky turned over to darkness, several rounds of fireworks burst through the sky, giving way to a full spectrum of magnificent colour. After the grand finale, Zandra and I began to make our way back to our hotel. The activities of the day had caught up with us. With full and joyful hearts, we wound our way back through the crowds, through a full lobby and bar, to our rooms. The eventful day had exhausted Zandra. She woke up and tested low several times throughout the night, requiring a lot of sugar to bring her levels back to normal.

The following day we planned a tour of the iconic Golden Circle, a tourist route into the southern uplands of Iceland. After an early morning and a quick breakfast, we walked to the day-tour building and boarded a coach bus to the UNESCO (United Nations Educational, Scientific and Cultural Organization) World Heritage Site of Vatnajökull. This beautiful valley is set between the North American and Eurasian tectonic plates and was a must in our planning guide. We were completely captivated by the expansive lava fields and crystal-clear streams throughout the area.

The next stop was at Gullfoss. The name Gullfoss translates to "Golden Falls." These falls are located in southwest Iceland and tumble down thirty-two metres over two stages. The first cascade is eleven metres and the second drops over twenty-one metres in a dramatic display that was completely awe-inspiring. In the summer, approximately 140 cubic metres of water rushes over the waterfall every second. As Zandra and I walked to the viewing decks, we were quickly soaked, then frozen by the sharp wind blowing through. The tourist shops offered local artisan woollen mittens, hats and scarves, but we found them to be nearly identical to what we already had in our shops at home, yet at a much steeper cost.

After the tour of Gullfoss, we boarded the bus and made our way to Geysir. The Haukadalur Valley is home to many geysers, some of which are rarely active and some that are more so. We were able to see shooting jets of boiling water up to forty metres high! The smaller geysers, like Strokkur, erupted every five to ten minutes and we were able to get a lot of photo opportunities of these in action. One of my favourite all-time photos of Zandra was at this tourist spot. The photo shows a girl, freely playing and anticipating one of the world's most exciting moments—a brief moment free from thoughts of blood sugars and insulin. Wherever we went, we had to account for how much insulin to bring, test strips and other supplies, as well as sugar and carbs. Even after several years of dealing with diabetes, forgetting something important was always a fear of mine. Zandra was in the age of hardly communicating with me, so I always used my best guess, never relying on her own estimations.

The burden of diabetes was ever present, so I took a moment to be fully in the present moment and enjoy our experience free of any worries—something I rarely did.

The following day was to be our last full one in Iceland. There was nothing more important for Zandra than to ride the infamous Icelandic horses; we had signed up for a riding tour before we came to Iceland to be sure that we made this one thing happen. Again we woke early, ate breakfast and headed to the tour operator down the road from our hotel. We boarded a chartered bus, rested into the comfortable luxury seats, and set out for the countryside.

As we drove along the country roads, I noticed how the views were markedly different from those of home. I could see steam being released from the ground along the rolling countryside, popping up along the dark black volcanic rock. Everywhere we looked, we could see what looked to us Canadians as campfires throughout the landscape. The steam percolated from the ground all around us and became a hallmark of our drive. This was something we didn't see in the Prairies! The drive was as enjoyable as each destination, and allowed us to see many beautiful farms and villages along the way. The bus brought us to a little farm in the middle of the rock and trees. We were greeted by members of a family and shown to the horses that we would be riding. The entire family, including the mother, father, son, and daughter, worked together to host guests and tour them across the countryside. They did their best to match horse with rider based on experience and size. I was given an old female horse that wasn't very interested in the thrill of a ride. Zandra was led to a horse whose name translated to "Guard," a young horse whose youth and energy were sure to keep up with the rider.

Icelandic horses are special because they are the only horse breed in the world that can perform five gaits, or ways of walking, while other horse breeds can only perform three or four. This information wasn't very exciting for me, but for Zandra, who loved riding lessons, she couldn't wait to feel the difference whilst on the back of a horse. The Icelandic horse is small, like our pony, but strong and stable. It has been a purebred in Iceland for over 1,000 years and strict regulations exist to preserve the lineage of the stock. No other type of horse is permitted in Iceland, so as not to interfere with these strict regulations. As an inexperienced rider, I didn't notice the differences riding this horse, but Zandra, as well as others in our group, were quick to point them out.

When we were set up on our horses and began to ride through the countryside, it didn't take long to get accustomed to the rhythm. The steady vibration of hooves trotting along the ground together with the gentle melodic sounds of nature allowed all the stress from the previous days to fade away. Although my horse wasn't interested in speed (and neither was I), we moved at a quick enough pace to keep things interesting. My horse treated me to a steady journey along the fjords that ran quite close to cliffs at times, which revealed the sounds and sights of waterfalls. At one point along our journey, we stopped for a break with our horses. We sat along the rocks, where refreshments were served, and rested in the shade. We tethered our horses and walked to the edge of the cliff where we could see the steep drop below us and feel the spray from the nearby falls. We were given the option to take a slower trail back or to pick up the pace and fast-track it. I immediately knew that Zandra would opt for the fast route, knowing that I wasn't advanced enough to follow her. I continued back separately from her, enjoying the remainder of the ride. As we separated, I watched her ride with confidence along the trail with the other faster riders. I felt so proud of her and her independent nature. The same personality traits that I was so often frustrated by were the same traits that I knew would see her through many future struggles.

The flight back to Canada went much more smoothly than the journey to Iceland. I was prepared with sugar in my purse this time, having learned my lesson. The airline unexpectedly moved us to first class to fill some vacant spots, which was a new experience for me as well as for Zandra. I often wondered how airlines made up in service for the price difference, and now I know. We were spoiled. We were handed warm, scented towels to wash our hands and were served several courses of delicious food that resembled nothing I'd ever eaten on a flight before. We had comfortable seats and our own folded-down TVs. The legroom was enough to justify the increased fare alone. We were given little bags filled with anything we could need: socks, toothbrush and paste, earphones, earplugs, etc. We flew home feeling like royalty. This was a trip of a lifetime for sure. We were home only a couple of days when we saw reports that the volcano that had threatened our trip had finally erupted, without causing much havoc at all.

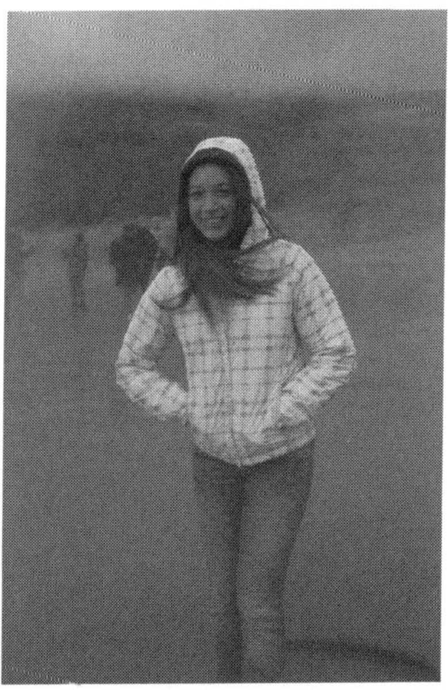

Zandra at the Geysir in Iceland

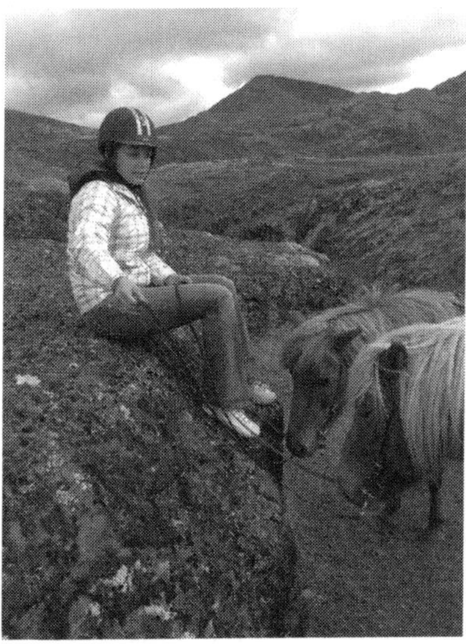

Zandra taking a break with the Icelandic horses

CHAPTER 8

Cinnamon

WHILE SCROLLING THROUGH TWITTER ONE day, I read a tweet from the Lions Foundation of Canada Dog Guides. They were starting up a new program for training diabetic-alert dogs and made the announcement to coincide with National Diabetes Awareness Day. They were promoting the program and asking for people who fit the criteria to apply. The timing was impeccable, as I had been investigating diabetic-alert dogs just days before and discovered that they were only available in the United States for a minimum of twenty thousand USD. A program that subsidized them was available, but only for US citizens. I had read articles about Canadians going across the border for these dogs and learned that they were worth their value, yet the price was far too much for us to consider.

I began researching anything I could find that would offset the impacts of Zandra's hypoglycemic unawareness. The truth was, I was scared and unable to sleep. Every night I feared that she would become low and not wake up. I would find myself at her bedside several times throughout the night, looking for the slightest movement of the blankets around her chest, reassured when I would see it. Oftentimes, I was too impatient or it was too dark to wait and notice, so I would give her a little tap to see if she responded. Zandra was a light sleeper, and on these occasions I would often unintentionally scare her awake.

I was less fearful of her daytime lows, because there were at least more people around her to assist her should she need help. The school administration and many staff knew she was diabetic and were helpful in any way they could be, although they weren't authorized to administer glucagon to a student, even though that's where she spent most of her time. As part of Zandra's medical supplies, we were given a prescription for a small case that included the hormone in a powder and a syringe filled with fluid. At the time of her diagnosis we were informed by the nurses that glucagon was a hormone made in the pancreas. It works with your liver to release stored glucose to your blood when there isn't enough in the bloodstream, and it needs to be injected in the event of severe hypoglycemia. I was grateful that the school was in close proximity to the hospital, should she be faced with an emergency. I felt comfortable that, whether she was at school or in sports, someone would help her access the help she needed. As Zandra got a bit older, we used the expired kits to teach her friends how to administer the glucagon by using a piece of fruit as the subject. I figured that if she was going to need it, one of her friends was likely to be around when she did—her group of girls loved her and were willing to do whatever it took to keep her safe. Although it hadn't happened, my greatest fear in the daytime was that she would go low too quickly and become unconscious.

My other frustration was that Zandra refused to wear her medic-alert bracelet. I had bought a bracelet and a necklace, both beautiful gold pieces that didn't resemble the generic drugstore-style jewellery. For her, they still looked like medically issued inventory and there was nothing I could say to her that changed her mind. When I would get angry, explaining that it could save her life on a bus, she would snap back, "I'd rather die," and end the conversation.

When I found the tweet, I knew it was a sign. What were the chances, after so much effort, to find such a lifeline? I immediately downloaded the link, read through the application form and printed it off. Although the application was long, I understood why. I was very aware of the value of the dog that we would receive, should we be accepted, and appreciated an organization that was cautious in screening their applicants. As an animal lover, I knew it was essential to be sure the home they were going into could support the needs of the animal. The application included a lengthy inquiry—name, address, phone, history with animals—as well as letters of recommendation from a veterinarian, friends, and from a medical specialist to substantiate the need for such a highly trained animal. I knew we could have all of these done quickly, and when we submitted the application, in my heart I was confident we would be approved.

The webpage indicated that, for the type of dog we were applying for, we couldn't have any other dogs in the home. After losing our beloved Murphy a week before diagnosis, it had taken my heart some time to heal before thinking of getting another one. I was beginning to feel ready to bring in another dog for our family, but this application was enough to stop any plans for a family dog in their tracks. When I questioned the trainers about our cats, they assured us that cats were not a problem. A diabetic-alert dog must always be working, even when not vested at home, so having another dog in the home is a distraction, as dogs work in packs and follow the alpha dog around. To maintain the order so the dog isn't confused, there must be no other dogs in the home, ensuring their person is always the alpha. Cats, we were told, aren't dominant and didn't pose a problem. Having two cats, I decided to agree to disagree with that statement. Our cat, Ma'at, always dominated Murphy, blocking his food dish or sitting on a stair so that he couldn't pass. Although the cat was only nine pounds and Murphy was sixty, there was an obvious power imbalance.

When Zandra came home from her soccer practice that evening, I spoke to her about a dog. She clearly didn't share my enthusiasm. She loved the idea of having her own dog, and knew that the dog would help her, but she had seen service dogs with their handlers in public and knew she didn't want that for herself. She agreed to only participate if she didn't have to take the dog to school. There wasn't any way she would be seen in public with a dog alerting the world to the fact that she had diabetes and needed help. I wasn't sure how exactly the dog worked, but I had a feeling that there would be an expectation to take her to school. We decided to go ahead and submit an application and follow the process. I hoped that in the time it took to meet a trainer she would have changed her mind.

A few months after our application was submitted, a trainer came from Oakville, Ontario to do a home visit. She was a petite lady with medium-brown, mid-length hair. She was small but confident, and it was clear that she had a lot of experience with the training and handling of guide dogs and their families. She wanted to check things off her list as far as our house and family members went, but also to screen us as applicants. She spoke with Gord and me, and with Zandra privately, about receiving a dog. When Zandra spoke about her apprehension, the trainer was clear that having a service dog meant not choosing when and where to take it. The trainer underscored this with, "All the dogs are fully trained to be companions wherever you go and have been training all their lives. In public, escalators, stores, work and school, the dogs know how to do their jobs." There was an expectation for the dog to go everywhere within reason, the exception being places they aren't safe and where it's not appropriate to have a dog, such as a professional kitchen. Otherwise, where she goes, the dog goes. This idea would take a lot of processing, as Zandra hated standing out in a crowd, but in the end she agreed to the terms.

The application took quite some time, as the training program was new and they needed a sufficient number of approved applicants-in-waiting. I was hoping that the time would help Zandra open up to the idea of having a dog and help her accept that she would be going to school with it. We were on the list for approximately eighteen months before we got the call to go to Oakville to train with her own dog. In the time that we had waited, nothing had really changed. The need for a dog was more pressing than ever, as the low blood sugars were still a daily struggle. Zandra was still resolute, however: determined not to show others that she needed help, still refusing to wear her medic-alert bracelet. Whenever I broached the subject, trying to get her to understand that I was feeling scared for a phone call that something had happened, or explained how I would head to her room each night and watch her breathe, I was told without any sympathy, "This isn't your disease and nobody asked you to worry." She clearly had no idea what it meant to be a mother, how every struggle she faced felt like my very own. There was no way for me to get her to understand that I wouldn't, even if I could, let her suffer alone. We were connected, even if this mother-daughter bond was understood by only one of us. No matter how much she pushed me away, I always loved her and would never stop.

I knew that there was no guarantee that the strength of my love ensured less suffering. I've realized that people don't get what they deserve; rather, they get what they need to evolve. I just prayed that my story, whatever it was, didn't end tragically.

The Lions Foundation paid for our tickets to Oakville so we could begin training. As Zandra was a minor, she required a parent to be present for the training and to be there for her should she need medical attention. I was quite excited to get the experience of both of us travelling to a city I had always wanted to see and to be amongst the amazing dogs at Dog Guides. This experienced humbled me in so many ways and offered hope for a situation that was causing so much distress in my life.

When we landed in Oakville, there were a couple of trainers wearing jackets with the telltale Dog Guides logos, holding signs with my and Zandra's names. It was the first time I had ever been greeted at an airport in this way but something I had seen countless times in the movies. I felt special. I was filled with nervous excitement and felt as though I could burst into tears at any moment. I appreciated that Gord was home with the other three kids, running their schedules and taking care of their needs for the nearly two weeks that I planned to be away. I understood what an extra burden this placed on a parent. Not only was I away for this time, I would be missing Olivia's thirteenth birthday as well as Mother's Day. I knew that they would all miss me, especially Olivia. Olivia was born on Mother's Day and was always a mommy's girl. She knew what this meant for her sister, but she knew what it meant to me, specifically. She has always been empathic in the same ways as me, and she required no explanation about the meaning of this trip. She graciously supported me in going, even if it meant being away on her special day.

After leaving the airport, we were shown to the large Dog Guides passenger van that was waiting outside. We were waiting on a few other people at arrive for other programs, so we got to meet and get to know the trainers while we waited. Each of the trainers proudly spoke of the facility and of their roles. We couldn't wait to meet the dog that they had selected for Zandra. A lot of effort goes into matching the right dog to each person, as a successful outcome requires the right relationship between handler and dog. We were told that we wouldn't be meeting the dog until several days into the training, when the handler was prepared to understand how to work with the dog.

The Dog Guides building resembled an old school. When we inquired about it, we were told it was in fact originally a school before it was converted for Dog Guides. The location was perfect, as it was in downtown Oakville, and we soon found that the walkability of the neighbourhood made it easy to access the places we needed. Oakville had an old charm and what looked like a rejuvenated downtown core. At that time, I worked for an organization that revitalized downtown areas and aimed to keep downtown economies thriving. I have always fully supported the "buy local" initiative, and, most importantly, allowing historic buildings to thrive through the generations. To me, this trip offered more than something to help Zandra, but also something special for me personally. After training in the day, we were encouraged to go out and check out the town. We just had to log in and out of the building for safety records. Zandra and I would often check out of the facility and walk for hours, enjoying the neighbourhoods and the opulence that spoke of old money. We could see the affluence in the yacht clubs that were nearby, and in the manicured landscapes around us.

We arrived a couple of days early for our training and were given the opportunity to see Niagara Falls. Oakville isn't far from Niagara, which was a place I had always wanted to see. One of the young trainers, Brittany, escorted us, along with the puppy that she was training at the time. It was a little farther than they would normally go, but it was a dream come true for us Albertans. Canada is such a large country that you can only truly appreciate it once you've travelled from one end to the other. Not only is it far in distance, but the climate is different in each region as well. We marvelled at all the differences along the trip, such as the trees being so much larger compared to ours at home. Everything seemed much more vibrant and green when contrasted with the prairie province that we had come from. Seeing the vastness of the open waters of Lake Ontario served as further reminder that we weren't in Alberta anymore. Until we arrived at Niagara Falls, I hadn't realized that Niagara itself was a city. I had assumed that the falls would be similar to the pull-over, side-of-the-road, sight-seeing attractions that were so familiar in the Rocky Mountains, perhaps with a few tourist shops and the usual smattering of restaurants and gas stations. I wondered how I never knew there was a thriving and beautiful city located here with all anyone could ask for, including what's called the Skylon Tower (a tower that looks like Seattle's Space Needle), soaring nearly 800 feet into the sky with a revolving dining room that rotates 360 degrees each hour.

We parked the van in the parking garage of an opulent building that overlooked the falls. It was a mall of sorts and something altogether unexpected. We walked along the road that led people to the viewpoints to see the falls. The walk through the city was a bit longer than what I had expected, but every bit as enjoyable with lush green spaces dotted here and there with picnic tables. There were large shade trees along the cliff that provided resting spots with a view. As we began to walk, the three of us with the puppy, I noticed Zandra beginning to walk slowly until she stumbled to the ground on the pavement. Her blood sugar had gone low and she hadn't noticed, probably due to the excitement and the walk that was taking longer than expected. We stopped and sat along the rock wall of a nearby restaurant that overlooked the falls. I pulled her tester out of my purse and she tested 2.3, much lower than the desired range of 4–8. I quickly inserted a straw into a juice box and passed it to her, with the full attention of the curious puppy at her feet. Moments like these were all too normal in our lives, but the normalcy never brought about an accepting heart. Every low that I watched Zandra manage hurt me, scarring my heart deeper and deeper in a way that nobody, not even Zandra, could see. This time, I felt a sense of relief that came from my new hope, that in future moments like this could be prevented.

Once Zandra's blood sugars were raised and she was feeling a bit better, we continued the walk to the viewpoints. We could hear the falls for a long while before we saw them come into full view. As we drew nearer, they became almost deafening. The falls were absolutely colossal compared to anything I had seen in Canada before. Images of the stunts that people have attempted in history—tight-roping across or going down in a barrel—flooded to my mind. I couldn't see how anyone could survive such a fall!

Tourist season was still a few weeks away, so all the boat tours for guests close to the famous Horseshoe Falls were closed, but that didn't matter to us. We were excited to be standing in view just the same.

From where we were, we could see the state of New York across the US-Canadian border, linked by what's called the Rainbow Bridge. I could clearly see the border stop and the thriving tourism industry on the other side.

After a quick walk along the viewpoints, Zandra and I separated from Brittany for a quick lunch before we had to set off back to Dog Guides. We found an interesting restaurant with outdoor seating on the upper level overlooking the downtown streets. We felt as if we were on a holiday, taking a break from the burdens that brought us to Ontario. We fully relished the moment, vowing to take opportunities not only on this trip, but in life, as you never know what you may be missing.

Our training was segregated into different programs. There was only one other lady who was there for a diabetic-alert dog. She was from Montreal and accompanied by her husband. She appeared to be in her late forties or early fifties. She was beautiful, with reddish hair and freckled skin, and she took great care of herself, as she not only looked amazing but she followed a healthy diet. She was there for the same reasons we were. Her blood sugars often fell dangerously low and sometimes she didn't wake up on her own, requiring someone to be there with a glucagon needle to revive her.

Meals were spent together, eating in the cafeteria or in the large lounge areas nearby. The facility trained dogs for many needs, including seizure alerts, hearing ears, service for those who are restricted with mobility, autism assistance, diabetic alerts and canine vision. With such a small diabetic-alert group, they placed us in tandem with the canine-vision class. We enjoyed our common time, including meals with the much larger class of seeing-eye dogs and their companions. The canine-vision class ran longer than the diabetic-alert program, so the day we arrived they were well underway and we were able watch when the participants received their new dogs. It was a heartwarming event to witness. It helped to cultivate our excitement for the dog we were going to soon meet.

Sitting down in the cafeteria for meals soon became a time both Zandra and I looked forward to. As a mother of four, I appreciated just being catered to. Every meal was served as customized by each individual. I didn't have any dietary restrictions, but Zandra was sure to let them know before she arrived that she didn't consume milk or wheat products.

The seeing-eye group was full of hilarious characters, and if it were a movie it would be a box-office hit for sure. An older gentleman, Terry, was a bachelor who lost his sight later in life. Although he was doing well by anyone's account, we could all tell he struggled. We could hear him banging into walls and doors throughout the hall and watched him clumsily drop his food at mealtimes, sometimes missing his mouth with his fork. He was a boisterous man who could sling the old boys' talk, telling tales of work trips and golfing tours. He seemed to appreciate his captive audience.

Polly, another seeing-eye client, had a gentleness that reminded me so much of my Nanna. She was soft and sweet and would never harm a soul. She too had lost her vision as an adult. She received a diagnosis about her failing vision in her early twenties and slowly lost sight until she lost her full vision in her forties. She shared stories of working for the government and of her independence in life, but seemed to take her vision loss in stride. The gratitude she had for her previous guide dog and best friend became evident in her tender stories. She had recently lost her canine companion to old age, but still required practical assistance as much as she needed a new best friend. Polly received her new dog, Poppy, and it was love at first pet for both dog and handler. They enjoyed retreating to their bedroom after our meals, no doubt for cuddling and quiet affection.

Rob was another client. He was from the Maritimes and was also receiving his second guide dog. Although he was very much a man of pride and strength, he didn't hold back tears when he told the group all about his old dog, who happened to be his best friend. He told the story of how he harnessed up his twelve-year-old cancer-ridden companion to lead him one last time into the vet clinic to be put down. The tenderness in his story had both Zandra and I silently crying as he spoke. Rob clearly loved his dog and owed his freedom to him. Although it was difficult, he knew he wanted and needed another dog. When he received his new service dog, he quickly noticed the personality differences from his old friend. He had clearly prepared himself for the anguish and newness of his new dog, and he expressed these differences as something that he was looking forward to getting to know in time. It was a wonderful experience to watch Rob and his new partner begin to establish a close new bond. Rob was one of those people who, like me, felt that animals were often more enlightened than humans. He appreciated his companion and never took him for granted.

One of the most comedic participants was a man named Jerry. He was in his mid-thirties and had been blind from birth. He was always smiling and up for an adventure. He had requested a Standard Poodle rather than the Labrador Retriever that everyone else in the group had. He had allergies, and luckily poodles are hypoallergenic. His poodle was highly intelligent and had a mischievous personality. If Jerry didn't have such an easygoing personality the match would have been doomed, but because he saw the hilarity of the dog they became a match that would provide endless entertainment. One afternoon while eating lunch, we watched the dog sneakily look around and slyly pop its head up to grab the other half of the sandwich on Jerry's plate, knowing that his master couldn't see. It was the funniest thing I had ever seen, but it was nevertheless a significant transgression for a service dog. A nearby trainer happened to watch the sandwich heist and quickly reprimanded the dog. Although we didn't see another sandwich get snatched, we regularly saw the dog looking to be naughty, and at times getting away with it. This pair could have their own reality-TV show!

One of my favourite dog guide recipients was a lady in her mid-forties named Sam. Both Zandra and I could sense her hard edge and knew that that lady was given challenges that attempted to knock her down in life. She had a chip on her shoulder that endeavoured to weigh her down, yet it motivated her to rise above it. Sam took an immediate liking to Zandra. She had a daughter of her own who was in university, something Sam was clearly very proud of. She shared with us that she had lost her vision when she was just a tot. Her mother's boyfriend had lost his temper in a drunken fit of rage and struck her across her head, leaving her with permanent vision loss. After that, she was removed from the home and grew up in foster care. I felt she had earned her tough edge. Sam was in a relationship with a man when she was younger and had a beautiful daughter from it before she again was jilted. Her daughter was her reason for wanting better for herself and something we bonded over as mothers. When she received her dog, those of us with vision could see the softness in her face. For those who couldn't see, they no doubt felt the love she kept safely guarded and now shared with her dog.

Not all dogs receive a perfect placement, at least not an obvious one. Amongst the older, more mature crowd was a young eighteen-year-old girl named Jennifer. Revealed in the way she spoke, her immaturity spoke to not only her age, but what I suspected was fetal-alcohol-spectrum disorder. She was loud, messy and very opinionated, but her youth afforded her leeway from me as she still had time to grow up. Also, she may have been nervous being away from her hometown of Fort McMurray. I was careful to avoid being too judgmental, as thoughts of myself as a child easily came to mind. I could hear my mom repeating the adage: "That's the pot calling the kettle black." So because of my own experience with Taffy, I couldn't judge.

Many of us, including myself and the other clients at Dog Guides, were concerned over the way Jennifer treated her dog, Zoe. We saw her pulling her dog along and not letting her lead, yelling at her and giving little affection. Jen had partial vision yet was legally blind. She was able to watch TV and text while holding the phone up very close to her nose, but she suffered from obvious vision loss, easily noticed by her scanning the room when speaking to her. Some of the other members of our group brought their concerns forward to the trainers. None of us wanted to see her go without a dog for support, but she needed to be shown how to treat a dog properly. From what I could see, she was offered extra support and training when the rest of us were off duty.

One evening at supper, all of us in the program were talking about the names of our dogs. Puppy litters are named alphabetically to easily identify the many different litters. One litter would all start with an "A" name, the next "B," and the one following, "C." The litters would go through the alphabet and repeat back at the beginning after a few years. After that, dogs are renamed, often by their donor, and their name can reflect the business or memorial of the donation. Many of the dogs that were trained for the canine-vision class were from the "Z" litter. Jennifer's dog, Zoe, was one of those dogs; however, she had been renamed. Jennifer explained to us at the dinner table that her dog's name was terrible before she requested—no, demanded—it be renamed to Zoe. When I asked what it was previously, she revealed that her dog's name was *Zandra*, and then continued to go on about what a terrible name it was and how she saved the dog from humiliation. Clearly she hadn't listened when we introduced ourselves and spoke as a group, otherwise I would hope she would have reined in her story. The rest of the group sat uncomfortably and went about eating their soup, unsure of how we may react.

Zandra and I could hardly contain our laughter, and we imagined that our friends who were visually impaired were glad to not have to awkwardly eye dart at one another while Jen went on and on. After the harangue, I loudly asked, "Please pass me the salad dressing, Zandra," and it was clear that Jen was oblivious.

Introducing a newly trained dog to its handler was what I imagined an arranged marriage might be: they don't know each other, what they look like or how they behave. For some people it was love at first sight, and for others the relationship would take some time, fostering a mutual respect and understanding that would hopefully develop into a deeper friendship and eventually love. For the unlucky, it would be a relationship that existed on tolerance. The excitement was building, knowing that somewhere, walking the halls, was Zandra's very own dog, and any day now we would meet him. We had absolutely no idea about the dog other than it would be a Lab—male or female, yellow or black, we didn't know. We got to work with other dogs while training, walking and doing basic skills, but not the one that would come home with us.

After a few days of learning how to handle and work with a service dog, the big day finally arrived. Not only was that moment exciting for Zandra and me, but the excitement was growing for the trainers. Each recipient was placed in their room to wait for the dog to come to their doors to be introduced. Each introduction would be personal and private, allowing for the bond to establish immediately and without expectation from onlookers. As Zandra and I waited in our shared room, I felt as excited as she did. Although I had been well schooled that I wasn't able to talk, pet or otherwise interact with this dog, I knew we would share a love for Zandra and both spend our lives dedicated to protecting and keeping her safe. It was a love that would be unique and promising . . . I couldn't wait.

When the moment finally came, the trainer knocked on the door. I opened it and an eager nose burst through. Even the dog knew this was a big moment, something to get excited about. When the yellow Lab came through, she immediately gravitated to Zandra, who had her hands outstretched and open. We were introduced to this beautiful dog, named Cinnamon. Many of the sponsors are from local groups as well as large corporations. Cinnamon was sponsored by a spice company, and as such they had the opportunity to rename her. She was in fact a dog that we had worked with the day prior, yet we hadn't known at the time she would be ours. Cinnamon and Zandra exchanged hugs and kisses, and spent the rest of the afternoon getting to know each other. Training between handler and dog would resume in the morning—they didn't want to place expectations on either, as the job of bonding was vital to the relationship. It was exceptionally hard for me to refrain from reaching a hand out to stroke Cinnamon's soft fur, but I had to resist. I needed this dog and didn't want to jeopardize the success between them.

Not all service dogs are encouraged to sleep on the bed with their handler, but diabetic-alert dogs are one exception. They can detect low blood sugars through the breath and sweat of the human, and being nearby means overnight lows can be caught more easily. We were warned, however, that every case is unique: some owners may not want dogs on their beds, nor did having the dog on the bed necessarily equate to better detection of nighttime lows. For the first night, Cinnamon was required to remain in her kennel, as it was familiar and safe for her in what is very much a stressful, albeit positive situation. I had never kennelled Murphy in all the years I had him; it always felt so cruel to me. I later realized that if I had, he may have been more comforted in storms and perhaps not have eaten everything in sight. During the training, I was able to observe new techniques and the reasons for them. I was beginning to open myself up to new ideas I had previously held strong judgment toward.

After spending time together before bed, Zandra walked Cinnamon to the concrete room, known as the "relief room," before kennelling her for the night. The room wasn't the most pleasant place to visit, as the stench from the dog urine and feces was overpowering. Even though it was cleaned and hosed down after each use, the smell still permeated the porous surfaces. Having Cinnamon was both thrilling and novel as she became a part of our family. For as much as Cinnamon was about to be a part of our family, I felt like a new stepparent: all the responsibility without any acknowledgement. As strange as I felt, I was just as elated as Zandra. We stayed in our beds reliving the day and accounting for all the cute things Cinnamon had already done in the short time we'd gotten to know her.

At some point in the night, we heard Cinnamon cry. We woke up and felt sorry for her being locked up and wondered if she was feeling stressed from the confines of her kennel, preferring to relax in the freedom of the open room. I wondered if kennel training was indeed too stringent—perhaps I was right to keep Murphy from one. I decided to reserve judgment until I had given it a chance. Zandra spoke softly to soothe Cinnamon, as softly as she could with a sleepy, groggy voice. She continued to reassure Cinnamon until we both fell back to sleep. A short time later we heard the whimpering again. This time I decided that she must need to relieve herself. Perhaps she had a nervous tummy. We were unfamiliar with this new dog, and I wondered if getting up every night was something we would have to prepare for. Zandra opened the kennel, comforted Cinnamon and walked her to the relieving room again. Zandra returned a short time later, frustrated that after walking all the way down a couple of long hallways, Cinnamon had just stood in the relief room without producing anything. She came back to the room, sent her back to the kennel and, remarkably, we both quickly returned to sleep despite these interruptions.

A short while later, we heard loud barks coming from the kennel. We were startled awake and surprised by the deep, unfamiliar bark. I felt as if I had a newborn baby again and didn't recognize their personality enough to perceive what sound matched the need. I was feeling frustrated, knowing that I likely wouldn't be able to return to sleep after this latest interruption. Zandra felt discouraged and inadequate. Things started to unravel for her and she began to cry. Through the muffled sounds of her snivelling she released the pent-up discourse she had been holding in. I appeased Zandra in the same ways I had done for myself all the times I dealt with an upset baby, until I could see the shift in her spirit. The mother in me wanted to take over the situation, to allow her to go back to sleep and manage Cinnamon on my own. I felt confident in my ability to take over and my instincts to do so were gnawing at me to make things right. Zandra took her new parental role as seriously as I did and immediately assumed responsibility for Cinnamon. As much as I could empathize with the feelings of inadequacy she was feeling, I had to let her experience them. The one thing I could do was support her. Unlike my own experiences, she wasn't alone. She slowly pulled her legs out of bed and shuffled to the kennel for the third time that night. She unlatched the kennel and let Cinnamon out. Cinnamon stopped barking but wouldn't stop pawing at Zandra. After a minute, Zandra decided she should test her blood sugar. The numbers on the tester read that she was low. It only took a moment before we were able to comprehend what was happening. Cinnamon was alerting her. Zandra pulled out a juice box and began to drink it while praising Cinnamon. I was in awe. Emotions began to flood my mind and overwhelm my senses. I began to shed silent tears as I watched Zandra sit cross-legged with Cinnamon peacefully collapsed on her lap. I had witnessed a miracle. We had no expectation that Cinnamon would alert before we even had a practice with her. Cinnamon had no experience alerting a "live low" until that night. I couldn't wait to share the news with Gord and the trainers in the morning. All the uncertainty I felt about getting a service dog quickly disappeared. I enjoyed the feeling of peaceful gratitude.

The following day, the new duo was up early and established a routine that would follow them for years to come. The sounds of the kibbles falling into the metal dish, the slosh of water as the dog filled her mouth and the sound of paws skittering along the floor were all signs of our new life. I woke with a sense of renewed confidence from our experience in the night. It was Mother's Day and I couldn't think of a better gift than having Cinnamon guarding over Zandra. Cinnamon knew her job well and was keen to practice.

That morning we worked with scent pods, which are filters that contain trapped breath samples from diabetic donors experiencing low blood sugar. Donors graciously supplied these samples after breathing into them, snapping on the medicine-cap-style lid and freezing them to preserve the breath. These pods were the tools to train the dogs and what they were familiar and confident with. Pods were the first encounter for the dogs before they work with live lows, even though we now knew Cinnamon was able to work very well with both.

Pods were placed on Zandra without Cinnamon noticing. Sometimes she put them in her pocket, sometimes she hid them in her hood. Once the scent pod lids were open, it only took a minute or two before Cinnamon caught on. Once Cinnamon detected the familiar scent of low blood sugar, the rest was a game to her. She immediately started wagging her tail and pawing at Zandra to tell her what she had discovered. Once Zandra was signalled, she was instructed to give Cinnamon a high-reward treat for a job well done.

Both diabetic-alert dogs in the program were excited to do their scent work. Cinnamon demonstrated already that she could work with live lows, but I could see that she loved and wanted to play with the pods. After working with scent pods, we practised "go get" and "go fetch," which essentially asks the dog to either go and get help or go and fetch a testing kit or juice box. All the dogs in the facility were trained to do basic work, but specialized where they needed to. I would never grow tired of watching dogs open doors, grab clothes from the dryer or open the fridge for a drink. Spending time surrounded by so many dogs felt like a place I could stay in. I didn't know how the experience would affect me, but I knew that I was right where I was supposed to be.

Once the basics were established, we quickly moved along to field trips. Our first field trip was at local coffee franchise just down the street. The trainer, Julie, set out with our other classmate and her companion and dog as well as Zandra, Cinnamon and me. The destination was only a few blocks away and served as a great first outing with the dogs. I could tell that Zandra was nervous. Whenever she was agitated, she became snippy with me and often rather rude. The walk was devolving by the minute as I trailed after Zandra, who ignored any effort I made to be positive.

Zandra walked down the sidewalk, careful to be walking Cinnamon in the ways that she was shown: on the left side with a little bit of slack in the lead. Whenever the dog was in public, she was fully vested and wearing her harness. This serves as a uniform that not only indicates to the public that the dog is working, but it's also for the dog's training. When in uniform, they know they cannot pull aside to relieve themselves or go off course sniffing around. The group practised pulling into a green space and taking the dogs off leash to allow them to relieve themselves before resuming our walk. Just this small action drew attention from onlookers and made Zandra uncomfortable. I could tell at that moment she was resistant.

Once we made it into the restaurant, we lined up for a coffee. There were several glances and audible *aws* from other people waiting in line. I saw how awkward it was in a lineup with Cinnamon, so I told Zandra that I would stay and she could find a seat. Just after we settled in our seats, Cinnamon let out a bark and captured the attention of everyone around. Zandra was immediately humiliated and upset, although she tried to hide it. The trainer was tuned in to what was happening and asked Zandra to wash her hands and test her blood sugars. Once she tested, it was obvious that Cinnamon was trying to again alert of low blood sugar. Ordinarily this would be a moment to celebrate, but I could tell that Zandra didn't feel that way. "Why did she bark and not paw at my leg like she did in practice?" she asked Julie. Julie responded, "She's learning how to communicate with you, so have some patience for both of you while you are learning." This response didn't quite appease the embarrassed teen but she survived it, and there would be many more moments to practice. The exhilaration from the first night had all but vanished.

That night, to celebrate Mother's Day we went out for dinner and a movie. We weren't able to go out alone with the dogs, so we left Cinnamon back in our room, secure in the kennel. Along our walk to the theatre we noticed an Indian restaurant and decided to enjoy a delicious curry. The movie theatre was only about a thirty-minute walk from the restaurant, so after our meal we headed out to find the theatre. We settled on watching *Woman in Gold*. The movie, starring Helen Mirren, was just what I needed. I felt like I teleported into the screen and drew strength from the determined and strong female lead. My thin veil of confidence was wearing thin and the movie offered me a recharge. I felt better able to step back into my own role and take charge.

A part of me was struggling as I tried to head off Zandra's snippets of frustration that she vented my way. I felt as if I was constantly treading water, trying to keep my head above each surprise wave. Staying positive through every frustration and fear was exhausting me. Whenever Zandra reacted with anger, I did my best to respond with encouragement and humour. It was taking its toll on me. I could see that the bond between Zandra and Cinnamon was healthy, but where I hoped that having Cinnamon would be enough to be open about her diabetes to work with her in public, I could see that it wasn't making the impact that I had prayed for.

In the months before we left for Ontario, Zandra had embarked on her first relationship with a boy. She was quite smitten and the excitement of this became a positive distraction when her life became difficult. Devin was in many of her classes and was also very athletic. They shared a mutual love of fitness and the outdoors. Neither one of them were lured by the typical rebellion of alcohol and late nights—these two would both rather be hiking or engaging in sports. They shared similar tastes in music and films, and spent a lot of time conversing about such topics. Devin was always curious about Zandra's diabetes and did his best to support her in any way he could. At the end of a long day, I could overhear Zandra relay the details about her training, including her frustrations with me, from our small quarters.

There were several more field trips that Zandra and I took part in while training in Oakville. Sometimes we grabbed a van full of other trainers and their dogs, and other times it was just the small diabetic-alert group. Julie was always fun to go out with. She genuinely wanted to see a successful match, and asked what stores and outings we were most likely to go to. We chose near-identical stores that we would ordinarily visit at home so we could become familiar with navigating them with Cinnamon. Each visit provided another opportunity to gain confidence and learn to navigate the shops as well as the other patrons. On one occasion, while we were walking through the furniture department of a Swedish furniture store, Zandra began to tire. She decided to sit down on one of the display sofas, which was covered with throw blankets and pillows. Cinnamon pulled up around the side of her to stay close and out of the way, as she was trained. While we were sitting, Cinnamon promptly placed her paw on Zandra to get her attention and alert her. Zandra pulled out her tester and realized that her fatigue was from low blood sugar. I had juice in my purse and handed it over to Zandra while she was pulling treats from her pocket to give to Cinnamon. This time was much better than the visit to the coffee shop, as Cinnamon alerted quietly without drawing attention from the other shoppers. This visit to the store resembled one that we would ordinarily do, but this time I had Cinnamon's help.

Field trips to the mall became the most memorable for me. A mall offers a lot of training opportunities for dogs, including escalators to navigate, walking through crowds of people, and food courts to practice the "leave it" command when they spot food on the floor. Zandra and I were free to roam across the mall by ourselves, and had planned to meet our group in an hour. We ended up going to a bathing suit shop, where Zandra found a new suit and learned to navigate a changing room with a dog, something I never imagined doing before this. It was so cute seeing a waggly tail popping outside of the curtained stall as she patiently watched Zandra change. When we had to stop at a restroom, Zandra hauled her into a stall and awkwardly realized that the wheelchair-access stalls were the only realistic option moving forward.

While we were walking on the second floor of the mall, we heard a big commotion. We walked to the railing where it overlooked the food court area and saw a woman yelling and rolling on the floor. We quickly noticed the large black Lab harnessed to her and watched him calmly hunker down while the trainer yelled and pulled away from the dog. It took me a moment to realize that what I was watching was a trainer and not a real incident. Once I realized this, I no longer felt like a shameful gawker, more like an interested observer. It was fascinating and something I had never expected to see. The trainer was working with a familiar dog from the facility named North, who was being trained in the autism-assistance program. She was putting the dog through a real-life episode of a meltdown in a mall. What struck Zandra and I both was how the trainer couldn't care less about what other people thought. Autism meltdowns were real and the rest of us just had to deal with it. My admiration for the trainers and their dogs grew tenfold in that moment. I also appreciated the opportunity for Zandra to see how trainers worked without caring what others thought. The moment was brilliant.

The best field trip was saved for last. Every dog and their handler were treated to a day in Toronto, to experience the city and learn to navigate their way in the world with their dogs. We were offered a choice to either take the train, which was something many of the seeing-eye dogs would be doing in their daily lives, or be driven. As we didn't see taking a train in our future, we opted for hitching a ride. Going to Toronto was a first for Zandra and me. I was a little intimidated, but excited at the same time. I packed my purse as usual, making sure that I had all that I needed in case of a low, before setting out. I was used to navigating my way through cities like Edmonton and Calgary, but Toronto was a city on a much larger scale. The highways were faster and bigger, and the sights were filled with historic elements mixed into modern roadways and buildings. I enjoyed being a passenger and not having to find my own way. We parked downtown, close to the famous Rogers Centre. It happened to be game day, and all we could see was a flood of blue trickling toward the stadium, crossing streets and roadways. It was exciting to be there just as the Blue Jays were getting ready to start.

We only had a few hours, so once we got outside, Zandra and I had to quickly decide where to go. The CN Tower was in view, but Zandra didn't have a burning desire to go there. We decided to walk over to the Ripley's Aquarium of Canada, and between the destination and the walk we would gain some experience being out and about with Cinnamon. Finding our way through downtown was a great way to immerse ourselves. We had to navigate around crosswalks and people, and look for green space to offer water to Cinnamon and relieve her. Zandra was getting quite proficient at unvesting Cinnamon before relieving her, although she clearly didn't feel comfortable. I loved the routines with Cinnamon, but Zandra did not. She felt very conspicuous to those around her. I tried my best to be lighthearted, but this was met with obvious frustration. Perhaps I was able to see things the way I did from my own exposure: having had four babies gave me a lot of opportunity to take myself less seriously. I no longer found changing diapers, spills and small disasters devastating. Perhaps I had become worn down like a rock in a river, losing the sharp edges that I once had. I had to allow Zandra to wear down her own sharp edges in her own time.

As we walked through the aquarium we captured a lot of glances, but it was overall a wonderful experience. Cinnamon was perfect and clearly looking to please her master. Zandra returned her efforts like a sharp-nosed head mistress. She was cognizant of what should constitute a working relationship in public, but I knew she would soften when out of the sight of the public.

After the aquarium, we continued to walk around downtown Toronto until we found Julie and the other couple in training. We were getting hungry and had come to a consensus that we would have lunch in a nearby Greek restaurant before heading home. The small restaurant was just off a main street, and offered a few round tables with chairs set out with a wrought-iron railing along the sidewalk for *al fresco* dining. Zandra and I went in and ordered our food. The employee offered us seating outside, which we preferred, so we walked out and waited for our meals to arrive. The other pair in the diabetic group preferred to stay in and dine. This option was met with resistance from the staff. They were told that they could not dine in with their dog. We were all very familiar through our training of the laws that allowed us access with the dogs, and taught to be prepared to handle some resistance, but nothing actually prepared us for being kicked out of a restaurant on our first big day. They were instructed to leave the premises, and the argument was drawing attention. Julie happened to be listening in and quickly came to their defence. She promptly pulled up the statute of law on her phone and showed them where it states the dogs were permitted access. She assured them that they were highly trained working dogs, but it was no use. It became clear that they either had to eat outside or leave. In the end, our friends decided to join us outside to avoid further hostility. Julie spoke of how to properly advocate with reason and fact. "You never win with shouting and arguing, rather with reason and follow-through." She said a win for Dog Guides is to follow up with a call and explain things when not in the heat of the moment. A public argument doesn't look good for the cause, even if they relent. Sometimes they could convince a reporter to write a news article, or a trouble-shooter could cover a story, but an all-out fight is never the goal.

When we returned to Dog Guides in Oakville, we met up with several of the trainees from the seeing-eye program. They were eager to hear of our adventures in Toronto, as they were awaiting their outing the following morning. We told them all about our adventures: where we went and how well Cinnamon and Zandra made out. We also mentioned the incident in the restaurant. They reacted to our experience with obvious disgust and frustration. Most of the group, having already learned the hard way to advocate and press for their needs, were indeed a group of rabble-rousers. When they came back the following day from their trip, they were pleased to report their choice for lunch. They had descended upon the Greek restaurant, a group of about eight dogs and their handlers, for lunch. The owners didn't dare confront this group of ready-to-resist patrons! I learned that people with disabilities could be some of the most bad-ass people out there.

The last night of the training ended with an annual appreciation banquet, which included dog recipients from the previous year to speak to their experiences, as well as a few new owners. Zandra was asked to speak about her experience and bravely went up to the front of the crowd of about forty people to say a few words. One of the speakers was the mother of a young boy who had received an autism assistance dog the year prior. She spoke of the difference the dog made in the life of her son, and her own in turn. She explained how at first the dog served to physically anchor her child, as he was a growing flight risk and had often run away into dangerous situations. Now, after learning he was tethered to a dog, the frequency of these attempts had almost completely ceased, and instead, when he felt overwhelmed, he just hugged or laid out on his dog. It was because of the dog that outings were even possible. She spoke of never being able to go to the dentist and having heart-wrenching experiences in the past where he had to be restrained while screaming and crying, but because of his dog he now felt comforted wherever he went. Listening to this mother speak from her heart about her son and his dog united us in an unspoken bond.

I knew how my own heart ached, and of all the silent tears that I shed through the love for my own children. The capacity to love until your heart aches so much that it feels as though it might burst is universal. All those days that I walked alongside Zandra, sharing her pain in a way that would never actually take it away from her, was such a burden, yet when I heard this mother express her gratitude for her son and his dog, I knew that she got it. She too understood. I suppose I knew this all along, but somehow my own struggles felt shared, as if a burden was lightened. Without knowing me, or my situation, this mother knew me and spoke directly to my heart.

The next day we were set to fly home. It was time to integrate Cinnamon into our world. We were nervous to fly with a dog for the first time but were assured Cinnamon would be just fine and would likely sleep on the plane for the way home. To be sure not to have any mishaps, we just needed to hold off on the meal and water closest to the flight, as we couldn't relieve her once we were in the airport or in the air. For those of us leaving that day, Julie walked us in and made sure we had the proper seats. We were told that whenever we booked our own seats, we had to make special arrangements for the dogs. By law, we had the right to do so. We were entitled to either an extra seat or a seat with extended floor room. We were cautioned that some airlines were more respectful of this than others and told to always advocate for ourselves. Just as Julie warned us, Guy and Nicole were told their extra seat was unavailable as the airline had oversold the flight. They weren't the type to cause a scene, but at the same time they needed the space. Julie jumped into action, having several heated arguments with the representatives they set in her way. She had the law on her side and demonstrated to us how to have a firm yet respectful argument. As she walked away with the extra ticket for the dog, we all silently cheered. At the same time, we hoped that we would never be put in the position to need to argue for a seat.

I noticed a lot of loving looks in both the airport and on the plane. To our surprise, the flight attendant, a middle-aged woman with a warm smile, approached us as we took to our seat. She told us that in her eyes, dogs are every bit as deserving of having their needs met, so all we had to do was call for help if we or Cinnamon needed anything. Cinnamon behaved very well during the four-hour flight home. The only time she was even noticed by the other passengers was when she started sleep-barking. Cinnamon let out a couple of fairly loud barks while her legs were going in full run, surprising all, especially the other passengers who hadn't noticed her sitting on the floor when they boarded the plane.

When we arrived home, all of the kids and Gord were excited to meet Cinnamon. Nobody was able to touch or acknowledge her, and Zandra was sure to uphold that rule. Cinnamon had to know who she worked for, and this meant not interacting with other family members. It was especially hard for the other kids, but, truth be told, for Gord and me as well. Cinnamon quickly learned her way around the house and yard. If she was stressed, it was hard to notice. Cinnamon was clearly an intelligent dog and, as I believe is the case with all animals, possesses a greater understanding of life than most people. She seemed to understand her role. I felt as though she understood that she was there to fill in where I wasn't able. She was to step in and take care of my baby, consoling her when she needed and protecting her from going to sleep and never waking up. I needed Cinnamon, and my appreciation and love for her was strong.

The first day of school with Cinnamon proved to be stressful for Zandra. As the only service dog at the school, seeing Cinnamon was exciting for her classmates and teachers. Zandra went from being inconspicuous to being fully exposed in a short time. Most people had no idea she was diabetic unless someone recalled the fundraising event for our trip to Iceland. She didn't want to raise flags that there was anything different about her or be thought of as weak. This fear was always her own, and one she projected to others. I could never see how anyone would perceive her to be weak or delicate, yet that was her fear. Now, with a service dog, it seemed to spell out "dependant." All of the confidence-building that had happened in Oakville seemed to disappear. Zandra quickly decided that she didn't want to take Cinnamon to school. Curious glances felt uncomfortable to her, which further spun into a negative inner dialogue. I had hoped and prayed that this wouldn't be the case, but no matter how much I wished it, it didn't happen, and I could see that we were in trouble.

The following day Zandra decided to leave Cinnamon at home from school. Nothing I could say or do would change her mind. I wanted to give it some time before I pulled the plug officially, as so much time and energy had been invested, not to mention that a living animal had crossed the country for her. I was heartbroken and couldn't get through to Zandra to change her stubborn decision.

When Cinnamon was left at home, I knew I wasn't supposed to interact with her, and did so as little as possible. While she was gone, Zandra wanted Cinnamon to stay in her room, which made for a very long day for her. I felt badly and let her outside for breaks midday. When Zandra returned from school, she would often find that her underwear had been eaten. This grew to be a daily occurrence, with Cinnamon knocking over the laundry hamper or going through a clean pile just for the underwear. This became expensive for me and frustrating for Zandra. My simple solution about putting laundry away and removing it from her room fell on deaf ears. I felt I was walking in a minefield, knowing that sooner or later there would be an explosion.

The trainers routinely check in on each dog and their partner to see how it's going, and a few weeks after we returned from Oakville they contacted us. It was clear to them that we were having some struggles. The trainer who came to follow up was explicit with Zandra that if Cinnamon was to work with her, she must go with her everywhere without exception. I was grateful for her clear boundaries. There was no mincing her words, and no room for debate. As for the underwear eating, the trainer explained that separation anxiety was likely the cause, and if Cinnamon were with her at school it would be prevented.

Things often seem to get worse before they got better. After the trainer laid out the rules, Zandra decided to ignore them. This continued for a couple of weeks, until one day, after leaving Cinnamon home again, we finally had it out—the bomb went off. With Cinnamon sitting beside a pile of newly chewed undies and frustrations mounting, I told her that I would not be party to keeping an unwanted dog. I was distressed and it was obvious. I couldn't keep back my anger and pain. I asked her point blank if she wanted to keep Cinnamon, to which she replied no. I told her that I would be contacting Dog Guides in the morning, and whatever the fallout we would deal with it. Zandra was indignant and retreated to her room with Cinnamon trailing behind. Even though Zandra was upset and hurt, I knew that she already loved Cinnamon and did her best to care for her. Cinnamon never lacked for love, attention, walks or care.

Later that evening, Zandra came to find me. Her face was swollen and wet with tears. It was clear that she had realized that I was serious about returning Cinnamon. She burst out in a new bout of tears and floods of emotion erupted from her. Long-held emotions from her diagnosis, her fears and her shyness were all pouring out in a torrent of sobs and tears. She begged me not to call Dog Guides. She pleaded that she didn't want to lose Cinnamon. She loved her and needed her, but had a hard time accepting her reality in view of the public. This was the moment I had been waiting for. I've always felt that acknowledging the truth leads a person to the goal, but unless the truth was revealed, one would always be lost and feeling stuck. This was Zandra's starting point. I hugged her and told her that it was going to all be okay. I reassured her that she wasn't alone or expected to be perfect, and that nobody, not even Dog Guides, believes in perfection. The next day Zandra left for school with Cinnamon following joyfully beside her.

Although the situation with Zandra and Cinnamon was improving, she was still experiencing difficulties at school. Her chemistry teacher had asked her to not bring Cinnamon to class. She explained that she had allergies to dogs and Cinnamon triggered them. Both Gord and I were oblivious to this new problem, as Zandra chose to deal with it herself. We noticed Zandra coming home to leave Cinnamon in a flurry between classes, then returning a couple of hours later to pick her up. When this became a pattern, we confronted her and asked what was happening. I was frustrated that there had been no communication with us by her or the teacher before being asked to remove her dog from class. "This isn't acceptable. There's a solution and I'm going to find one," I said.

"Please don't call. Let me handle this on my own," Zandra insisted. I decided to give her the opportunity to explore solutions on her own; however, she had to keep me in the loop.

Giving Zandra the freedom to solve her own problems meant letting go and giving her the space to do so. This was a test for me. The solution made by the teacher was to place Cinnamon in the infirmary room of the school office while chemistry class was in session. It was only a few days into this arrangement before Zandra went to retrieve Cinnamon and found her playing with another student who was sitting in the office. After that, Cinnamon was placed in the library, where there was a spot for her to stay. As it happened, no classes were coming in during that block. Soon after the move to the library, the janitor complained about the dog fur accumulating on the carpet. Cinnamon had to find another place to be for chemistry class. The problem was brought up with the principal and his suggestion was to place Cinnamon in the custodian's closet with the mops and cleaning products. When Zandra told me of this, I could no longer stay silent. I needed to set up a meeting with the teacher and principal straight away.

I called the school secretary, whom I've always enjoyed talking to, and she set up a meeting for the following day after school. When Zandra transferred to the school in Grade 8, Pat, the principal, was so lovely that he made me want to be in high school again. Pat had recently retired and a new principal had transferred into that role.

I went into the meeting frustrated, but open to hearing other points of view. I arrived at the school just a few minutes prior to the meeting time. I glanced down the hall and saw the principal approaching. Our eyes met quickly before he darted away into an office down the hall. I got the sense he felt awkward, as he knew why I was there. I walked down the hall and located Zandra coming my way. We were immediately escorted to the boardroom to wait for the teacher and principal to arrive. Soon after, the teacher came in and introduced herself. She came across as quite pleasant, so I can see how Zandra wanted to please her. We all sat together for a few minutes to wait for the principal to join us. We waited another ten minutes until the teacher went to have him paged by the secretary. He was reportedly still in the school and had been reminded of our appointment. We continued to wait for another fifteen minutes until it was clear that he wasn't coming. The three of us decided to commence the meeting and find a solution. Zandra's teacher said she felt uncomfortable with the principal's proposal to have Cinnamon stay in the cleaning room and knew we had run out of options. I explained that legally we had a right to be there, but in no way wanted to create a problem with her allergies. After just a couple of minutes, we all agreed on a solution: Zandra would sit toward the back of the class with Cinnamon. If she needed to come forward, she would keep Cinnamon at her desk while she approached the front of the class. This was a resolution that we all found agreeable. I had my suspicions that her concern with Cinnamon was more to do with fear than allergies, but even so, with open minds and communication, we found a way forward.

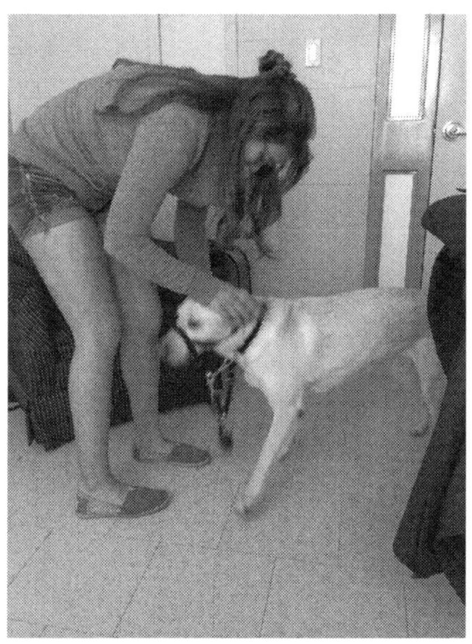

Zandra meeting Cinnamon for the first time

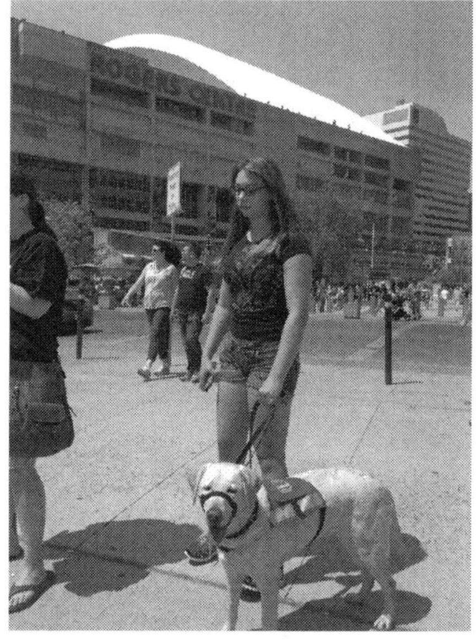

Zandra strolling with Cinnamon in Toronto

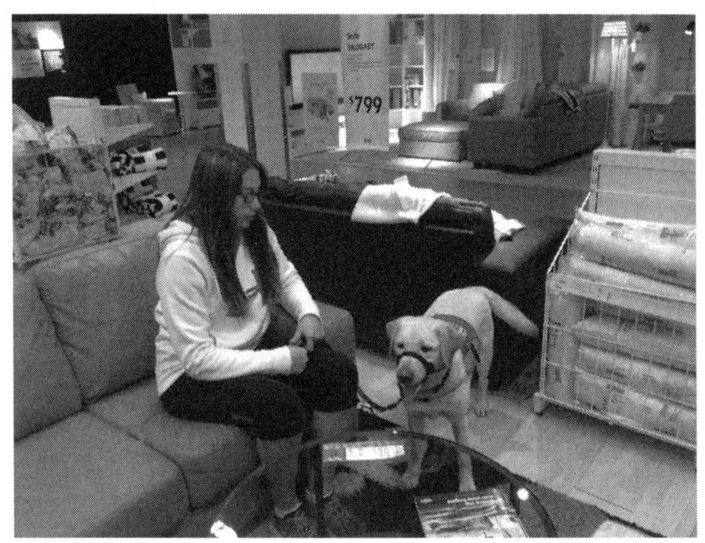

Zandra experiencing low blood sugar while shopping with Cinnamon by her side

CHAPTER 9

No Longer a Child

NO MATTER WHERE YOU GO, "child" is defined differently. We often think of a child as anyone under the age of majority. When you fly with an airline, for example, a child is anyone under the age of thirteen. The age that children are phased out of the Stollery Children's Hospital is seventeen, which meant that at age sixteen we were being transitioned out. When I was newly eighteen I was already moved out on my own, navigating my way through the world. I was resourceful and determined but, in ways that I never saw, I was also naive and reckless. I didn't have parents present who were looking out for me, guiding me through decisions and explaining my options. I grew up, like many my age, in the school of hard knocks. At some point in my years of parenting, my perspective shifted. As a parent, I see how childlike an eighteen-year-old is, not to mention a sixteen- or seventeen-year-old.

Neuroscientists generally agree that our brains haven't fully developed until around age twenty-five. Before then, the frontal lobe, which helps us be fully aware in decision making, hasn't even fully formed! So, when the Stollery indicated that at age sixteen they were preparing us for leaving, my heart hurt. I felt as though the science wasn't consistent. These kids needed the oversight of their network of doctors and nurses that they have known for their journey through diabetes. My child wasn't ready. I wasn't ready. I couldn't bear the thought of being cast out of a place that provided comfort and stability, especially during the teenage years.

Life felt like it was happening too fast, as though I was on a busy bus that was moving quickly through the streets and I had to have my wits about me so I didn't miss my stop. I suddenly had to prepare myself for Zandra's release into the world. Zandra's nurses were my way of understanding what was happening with my daughter. They had become my sounding board and had in a large way co-parented Zandra and supported us through many rough waters. I felt like I was being abandoned to make way for someone else. My heart began grieving the loss before it even happened.

We were told that there was an adult clinic that was nearby; however, it was structured differently as their patients were adults of varying ages. The same type of care couldn't be expected any longer. It was suggested that if Zandra had any plans to consider pump therapy, we had to act quickly. There was a waiting list for classes, and if we were added to the list immediately we might just make it before we were out of the clinic. Zandra seemed to understand that this was her best chance for training on a new system and reluctantly decided to go on the list. She was apprehensive to change from her multiple daily injections to a pump, but she knew that if she were to change, this was the time and place to do it. She could easily recall the struggles she'd had the last time she gave the pump a chance, yet she understood that the specialized care at the Stollery was as good as it gets, so she inched forward toward adulting.

When the classes started, Zandra was the oldest patient there. The sessions were held in a training room of the hospital, which looked like a mini lecture room, with the floor being on multiple levels toward the back of the space. Everyone was provided a desk with a good view of the screen, and the presenters were at the front.

The children in the class ranged in age from toddlers to teens and the class was full. The trainers included a nurse from the clinic and a dietician, who wore a pump herself to manage her own diabetes. From the very beginning of the class, Zandra took over her training. She seemed bothered that I showed an interest when I would likely never have to operate her pump on my own. She seemed set to exclude me in the training, preferring me to be more of a chauffeur and lunchmate then the caregiver I was.

Every other parent in the room participated in learning how to set basal doses, which are micro-doses of insulin that are continually administered through the pump site. There was so much to setting and changing these rates that I was quickly overwhelmed and inwardly relieved that I could take a more supportive role rather than the others, who had to crunch the numbers. I thought I knew a lot going into the class—I understood hormones that affect blood sugars and how different types of foods interfere with absorption of insulin—but there's always a lot more to learn. The saying, 'The more you learn, the less you know," had never been truer.

I had always been a hands-on parent until we started pump class. Zandra was clear that I would never be wearing her pump and would never need to know how it worked. I felt frustration and rejection, but this time I had to prepare myself that things were changing. Soon I wouldn't have the team behind me that understood the teenage rebellion I was seeing at home. I would be without the indirect narrative and eye glances that her doctors and nurses had become so fluent in. I had to change. I had to accept that I was nothing more than support, if I was ever anything else. Zandra was right: this wasn't my disease, but I still didn't feel I had an official place.

As classes continued, I sat back and watched. Whenever the parents were prompted to set the pumps for the class scenarios, I sat like a lump and watched Zandra do it on her own. I had to grieve that for the first time I wouldn't help with this. The pump was confusing and much harder than I thought it would be. I highly respected and admired the parents of young children who were in the trenches and acting as caregivers. I would have been one of those parents who learned the pump inside out for the benefit of their child, but my role was changing. I was being sent into a forced retirement, having to submit to a new role, unsure of what that looked like.

I had to change gears and be more of an encourager and less of a caregiver. I had to be on the sidelines and let her learn from the same school of hard knocks that had taught me. I had to accept whatever fate was before me and trust that Zandra had learned alongside me during the last five years. I realized that I had to define my own role from that moment forward so I could offer whatever assistance I could without unrealistic expectations placed on either of us. I needed to realize that my role was not to prevent mistakes, but to support learning from them. My fear of failure had been passed down to her. As I watched her work through her numbers, I could see her frustration when she miscalculated a number or missed a step. I recognized the immediate rejection she took to heart whenever something went wrong. In that moment, I could see that I needed to teach her something that I was only beginning to understand myself: she needed to learn how to fail.

The insulin pump had been well recommended by all of our diabetic friends, nurses and doctors. Everyone on the pump professed to the freedom it provided and said they would never go back to needles again, despite the frustration of operating the pump. In the time that lapsed from our first encounter with the pump to the classes, the province of Alberta had adopted a plan that covered the cost of the pump itself, which was just less than seven thousand dollars. This made the decision to transition much easier, although the cost of the supplies was still borne by the user. Thankfully, given our family's medical plans, we've always had most of our costs covered.

A representative came to our house to show us the pump in more detail and answer any questions we had. There were a few models to choose from, depending on Zandra's needs, but the one we chose came highly recommended by everyone. We heard how a friend was travelling in Europe when her pump failed and she had to go on needles at the last minute. This company promises to supply pumps anywhere in the world within twenty-four hours, and our friend was a testimony to the company upholding its promise. Each style offered something different, and although there were only a few models to choose from, the brand we chose was Zandra's final choice, thanks to the personal experiences of those we knew.

Wearing an insulin pump came with its own challenges. The injection site needed to be changed every couple of days. This wasn't unlike giving needles. Every time the needle was replaced it needed to be on fresh skin to avoid lipodystrophy—an abnormal accumulation of fat tissue causing the dreaded "lump." This lump can interfere with absorption of the insulin and create additional problems to the person with diabetes. When Zandra was first diagnosed, we were given a diagram that was, in essence, a map of where on the body to inject and how to rotate the injection site to avoid reusing the same spots. In the end, each user found their favourite places and did their best to rotate and switch them up as needed.

Zandra never formed lumps of significant size, but there were times where some were beginning to appear and she needed to be mindful of them. It seemed to happen so quickly that it was always a surprise to me. Zandra would notice, yet never tell me at home. I always found out during discussions with her doctors and nurses. A few months without using the site would usually clear them up, but every time I saw a side effect reveal itself on her it wounded a part of me. It was a reminder that I couldn't protect her and keep her safe from everything. Even a rather innocuous lump was able to hurt the secret place within me that held all my own wounds. I understood that the day would come where there would be a day of reckoning with all the hurts that I kept under lock and key, but not until I was ready.

The infusion site where the needle with the insulin tube is inserted has a couple of options: straight or curved needles. Both were very uncomfortable for Zandra. She was very lean and didn't have a lot for a needle to go through, and they had to be held with tape for a couple of days at a time. Although I sympathized with her, I was always very appreciative that she was sixteen and not six or younger. I couldn't imagine setting an infusion site to the sparrow-like arm of a three-year-old, yet parents all over the globe have to face that reality, if they're lucky enough to be afforded a pump.

As much as Zandra had a change of heart about receiving a pump, I realized that there were layers of acceptance that she had to work through, ones that I couldn't really understand. I'm sure that as a teenager with a boyfriend she had concerns about how she would look and feel, especially when thinking of being caressed or in a moment of closeness. I'm sure she wondered if the tubes coming from her body or the cumbersome pump itself would be a barrier or a turn-off to someone else. Fortunately, Devin, who was still a part of her life, didn't seem to care. Moreover, he seemed very intrigued about the pump and how it worked.

The pump classes were very comprehensive, and after having the pump for several weeks, Zandra was glad she went through with it. She struggled for a while with how to wear the pump to bed and how to conceal it under clothes, but I noticed that the more she wore it, the less she cared about hiding it. It became an extension of her, much like an arm or a leg. In the same way that a wheelchair becomes an extension of someone who relies on it for their mobility—so much so that anyone touching their chair can become offensive and require consent—so too was Zandra with her pump. It was personal, yet she began to accept it as a part of herself.

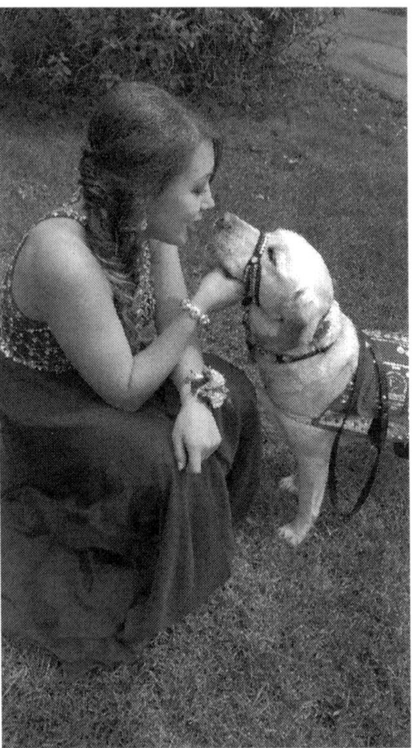

High School graduation

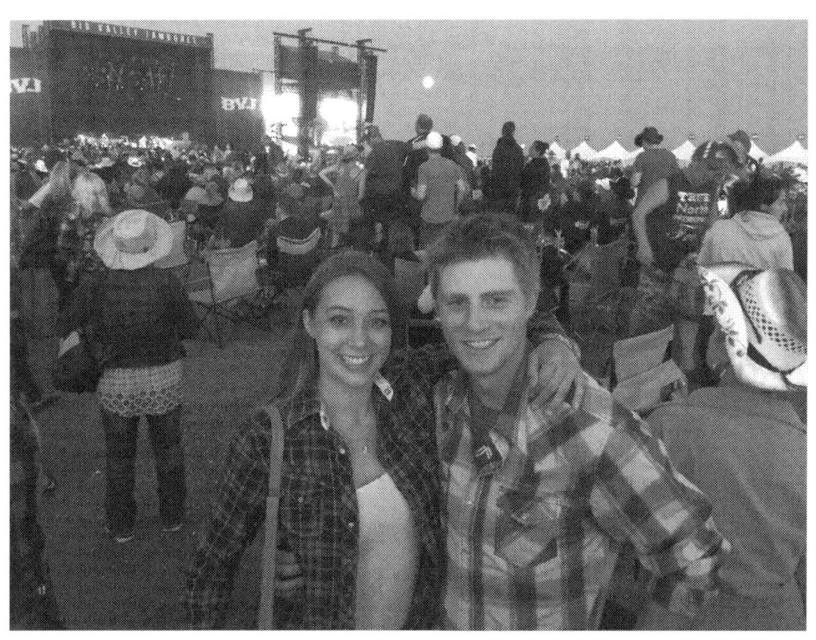

Zandra and Devin at Big Valley Jamboree

CHAPTER 10

University Bound

"I KNOW EXACTLY WHAT I WANT to do," Zandra emphatically told us. "I'm going to pursue dietetics at the University of Alberta." When Zandra decided to do something, she was most often resolute. So when she gained acceptance into her program of choice, we immediately turned our minds to the upcoming move. Edmonton was only an hour away from home and her move there would have her even closer to her aunties, uncles and cousins living in the city. I felt quite comfortable with her flying the coop, even though she was only seventeen.

The dietetics program was a natural fit for Zandra. She had turned to veganism at the beginning of high school and had adhered to it quite strictly despite all the peer pressure she faced. From childhood, she had been avoiding many foods out of necessity, and since her diagnosis she had looked at food as a tool to help her gain control of her health. To her, food could heal or harm, and if she had a chance to limit the impact of her diabetes she was going to do it. At first, she noticed a positive change with her blood sugars—her levels became more stable and she was feeling great, but this honeymoon period wasn't to last. After the first year, she was disheartened. Any lowering of insulin had soon rebounded and the result in the end was no different than it was before she became a vegan.

I imagined her daydreams matched mine: ever hopeful that a simple cure lay just outside of our understanding, ready to be discovered. Ever hopeful that a change of diet would be the cure, yet not wanting to say it out loud for fear of looking foolish and being taken in by a fad. In my daydream I could see the smiling face of my daughter as all of her hard work and struggles paid off in the end. Zandra's determination gave me hope. Although I knew that if diet was the answer it likely would have been discovered before, her sheer power of will offered me something to hope for, with its childlike reverie.

Zandra worked hard and stayed on course to make the changes in her diet. I stood by and felt the excitement when she would announce good blood sugars with less insulin, yet as time went on the changes were insignificant. She was determined to stick with it, despite feeling betrayed by her own body. She believed in the healing power of a clean diet and she wanted to learn more. She wanted to combine her love of science with her powerful determination and belief that food held value in healing to prove to the world that a cure is out there and that changing your diet is the first step. The dietetics program matched her seventeen-year-old ideals. She was excited to learn about nutrition through a scientific lens, and going to university would align her heart and mind.

Having Cinnamon around meant looking for living accommodations that offered some green space nearby, as well as a lifestyle that suited them both. Zandra was never into the party scene; she liked the quiet life with some good friends she could call upon to fill the need to socialize. Both she and Devin were more introverted by nature, and the idea of moving into university residency was quickly struck from the list of options. Both Gord and I felt that, as her plan was to live in Edmonton for the next several years, it was an opportunity to purchase a small condo that had the potential to make some money down the road. The benefit of this option was that we wouldn't have the hassle of landlords and we could be choosy about her living arrangements.

We looked at a lot of housing options but ended up settling on a condominium, appropriately named University House. It was a short walk from the campus and featured a nice-looking '80s style four-storey walk-up. The suite had modern updates and two bedrooms. It was on the main floor with a small green space outside the patio doors that offered Cinnamon a place to easily relieve herself without Zandra having to go for a walk down the Whyte Avenue area of Edmonton alone. At first we weren't sure about a main-floor suite, but quickly saw the benefits of not having to juggle flights of stairs with books, bikes and groceries.

It didn't take long until we found a perfect roommate. Tori was a family friend who was in her early twenties and working on her master's in engineering, and we knew she would be the perfect roommate. She had lived independently from her family for several years and was very social. My worry was that Zandra would shut herself away and not enjoy university life, and Tori became the perfect balance.

So many parents looked to rein in their teens from excessive partying and staying out, but for Zandra it was quite the opposite. Isolation could be just as stressful and threaten her success at school. Tori was exceptionally bright and easy to talk to. She made friends wherever she went and I knew this was just what Zandra needed. Tori also grew up with her mom being a type 1 diabetic, and as such understood the nature of the disease. She knew what to do if Zandra experienced a dangerous low. Her presence was to be a great comfort to me.

My greatest fear was always the nighttime lows. I had become accustomed to peeking in on Zandra through the nights. Watching and listening to her breathing gave me a comfort that I was no longer able to have. I needed this reassurance for my own peace of mind and rest. Soon I would have to leave my role of night watcher and learn to live without it. As much as I wanted to express my worry to Zandra, Gord, or anyone, I realized how alone I was. The words would catch in my throat like a ball that refused to budge. They were caught in a place that was scared to admit the worst for fear that it could come true. I didn't want to worry Zandra either. She had done the hard part. She had studied so hard to earn her place in the program and I knew full well that placing fear with her would be as destructive as giving her poison. Instead of telling her my fears, I moved toward positive reinforcement, more for her benefit than mine. "I'm so glad to know that you pay such close attention to your health that I can rest assured you'll be just fine." I didn't know if this isolated her further, but it was better than telling her I was scared that one night she would never wake up.

Having Cinnamon by her side had always given me comfort, but she didn't always catch the nighttime lows. There's never a guarantee that a service dog will catch all lows, but nighttime ones were always an extra gamble. Cinnamon was a special tool but could never be solely responsible for preventing a severe low. A tired dog can sleep through anything, just the same as a person. I also couldn't ask Tori to stand in for me and look in on her every night, even if Zandra would allow it—which she wouldn't. I needed faith. I had to lean on a higher power than myself. I turned to God every night. I prayed that He would send angels to watch over her and keep her safe. I never liked praying this prayer. It meant that by my asking, I was acknowledging that things could go desperately wrong. I prayed that, should things indeed go wrong, Zandra would be surrounded by those angels as well as having Cinnamon by her side. The prayer I would often recite as a child before bed came to mind:

Now I lay me down to sleep,
I pray the Lord my soul to keep.
If I should die before I wake,
I pray the Lord my soul to take.

My comfort was always knowing that, whatever happened, she wouldn't be alone.

As the first day of school was approaching, Zandra was busy getting familiar with the website for the university. She saw that the faculty provided an orientation for the new students the day before classes commenced and immediately knew this could help alleviate some of her stress on the first day. She had called me to let me know and was quite relieved, as it was such a large campus and she had no idea where to go. She had told me that she had found the place where the tour started, so at least she knew how long it would take to make it on time and where to meet the others. The next day she called me crying. It turned out that students had to sign up online for the tour, as they only took a limited number. As she stood holding Cinnamon's leash, she was told she couldn't join at the last minute. Zandra felt completely embarrassed and foolish. She chastised herself for not understanding that she needed to sign up. I tried to explain to her that it wasn't stupidity, just naivety, but the rejection was felt deeper than my words could reach. I understood her shame and wanted desperately to make it better. Both Gord and I offered to walk with her to find where she needed to go, but in the end, James, my brother-in-law who lived nearby, offered to take her instead. He knew the campus much better than we did, as he was the last in the family to graduate. That day he picked her up and walked her through the campus, finding all of the buildings she would need to be familiar with. They toured the bookstore, the library, and the HUB (housing union building) mall with all the fast food and coffee options, as well as proximity to her condo. I was eternally grateful to James, and so was Zandra. Although she was still nervous, she at least had an idea where things were.

Zandra was keen on finding her own way. Her tendency was to be harsh with herself when something didn't go as planned. She revealed to me that this was her way of being sure that she wouldn't make the same mistake again. I was recognizing this trait more and more with her and knew from experience that it could lead down a sad and lonely road. She convinced herself that to see positive results she needed to be fully scorned, so she took the job of punishing herself for her mistakes, for every oversight that could have been prevented, in earnest.

While planning her first-semester courses, Zandra was ambitious and filled her timetable with challenging classes, including chemistry, stats, math and extra science labs. She had a full schedule ahead of her. When her class schedule was set, some of her days during the week began at eight o'clock in the morning and didn't end until nine at night. The class schedule seemed onerous, but she insisted she could handle it.

Zandra called me after her first chemistry class. She was sobbing so hard it was difficult to make out what was wrong. I was standing in the living room trying to quickly turn up the volume on my phone to hear through her intense emotion. I was able to calm her down enough to hear her words more distinctly. She was clearly feeling hopeless. "I didn't understand what the professor was teaching. I had never heard it before, so when I went to see him after class he told me that it was Grade 12 work and if I didn't know it by now I wouldn't pass his class." Zandra was a very keen chemistry student, and if it was in her Grade 12 curriculum, she would have remembered it. I told her that some professors gave the tough-guy act to test the thickness of their skin. I told her that I had every reason to believe that she would do very well, but she did have to learn to get a thick skin. The only way to do that was to experience the heat of the scorn and respond with positive self-talk. I felt like a hypocrite. Although I've been at the receiving end of a lot of criticism, I knew that every word left an invisible scar. I still felt every shameful word ever said to me in the pain room I held deep within me. Although I had done a lot of work to move through my own shame and inadequacy, I still had a lot of unresolved grief. I felt like an imposter doling out advice and realized that it was time for me to heed it for myself. As I led Zandra through healing affirmations, I was walking my own path, sorting out my own room and learning how to let go. I prayed that she would fare better at the young-adult boot camp than I had.

My grief was as old as I was, grief that ran as deep as my veins from my earliest childhood memories. I felt as though I didn't have anyone there for me to guide me through those years, but I would be damned if I let my daughter feel as alone as I did. I felt as though the spotlight was on me, and now more than ever I had to step up and practice what I was preaching. I had to be the change I wanted to see in her. In my heart I knew that this journey would release the chains that bound me. In a compelling and beautiful way, I was being gifted the opportunity to revisit and heal myself by helping her. With every suggestion and piece of advice I had, I questioned my own ability to live that practice in my own life. More often than not, I had to work extra hard to change well-practised patterns of my own. I owed it to the next in line. I wanted Liv, Joseph and Liam to see a living example of how to forgive oneself and live a life in playfulness and wonder, rather than piling on the burdens and harshness of reality, creating a hardened shell.

Every class became a struggle for Zandra. One Saturday she called me from the school where she was in a long lineup of students waiting for a chance to receive extra help. She was upset because the line was hours long and one of the boys in the line ahead of her was throwing up in a bucket that he was holding. When Zandra asked if he was sick, he responded, "No, I'm just anxious." It appeared that she wasn't the only one who was having difficulty or feeling stressed. Zandra had always had a weak stomach and was never able to handle the smell of vomit, much less the sight. As she was waiting in line, she was feeling herself growing ill as well. Fortunately for her, the student could no longer continue waiting and pulled himself from the line before he had the chance to seek help.

As the first couple of months passed, I had hoped that the stress of school would subside, and that she would settle into routine that allowed for fun and lighthearted calls, but I was wrong. I continued getting near daily calls of crying and low confidence. These calls were taking a toll on me as well. I was worried and felt her pain as my own. Although she came home on weekends, leaving the house on Sunday evenings was difficult for us both. Sending her off into the stress where she wasn't thriving grew increasingly difficult for me. Both Gord and I wondered if university was in fact the best option for her. Even Tori noticed that the distress often felt by a new student wasn't fading for Zandra as it normally does for new students. She tried her best to include her in activities and comfort her, but felt it was making little difference as well.

The stress was not only taking a toll emotionally, but also physically. Zandra had an upcoming appointment with the adult diabetes clinic in Edmonton. I wasn't able to go with her, but as it wasn't too far for her to walk, she went alone. I planned to touch base with her after her appointment to see how things had gone. Normally the appointments consisted of monitoring bloodwork as well as making any pump adjustments that were required.

About an hour after her appointment, she called me. I could hear the traffic from the cars in the busy university area idling by, as well as her footsteps in the snow. I heard sobbing, but wondered if somehow I had caught a pocket dial, as nobody was speaking on the other end. I called out her name so she was aware I was on the other end and continued to wait. I was about to end the call when I heard a faint "Mom" from the other end. The grief in her voice sent a terrible shiver through my body. I immediately knew something was wrong and prepared as best as I could in the moment to hear what she had to say. She could barely speak the words but managed to sputter them out between what I could tell was a combination of weeping and panic. She struggled to tell me that in addition to diabetes, she was diagnosed with thyroid disease, more specifically Hashimoto's thyroiditis. She said her A1C was higher than ever and could be affected by the underactive thyroid. The word *disease* triggered her panic and she had begun spiralling. She was given a prescription to offset her underactive thyroid and told that she would need to take it daily for life. She wasn't able to recall anything else from the visit.

I desperately wished I were there with her. I had a lot of questions and regretted that I hadn't cleared my schedule to make sure I was present to support her. I told her I would come immediately, but she said she had a full day of classes and needed to head straight to school. I tried to console her by reminding her of my own diagnosis of thyroid disease and how it was something I could live with and manage with the same medication she was prescribed. My words seemed to make little difference. In her state, she felt entirely defeated. She berated herself and her body for not functioning properly. She felt utterly betrayed by her body. She had worked so hard to manage her diabetes—eating a vegan diet and working out to stay healthy—only for it to respond with yet another disease. She felt hopeless and wanted to throw in the towel. I tried to assure her that in every step, God was with her and she wasn't in it alone for a minute. I assured her that He must have very special plans for her that she's had so many struggles. She was being trained to be strong and there were lessons in this that she needed to learn to evolve her spirit. I was grasping. In truth, I wondered the very same things. Although I knew there were parents in hospitals all around us who questioned the universe why their child was ill, this was *my* child. I too felt alone and scared. I was tired and wanted her pain to end. I envied the photos on Facebook of her classmates loving university life and living it to the fullest. I would have given anything for the same experience for Zandra.

Every day I made sure to send Zandra a daily quote from one of her favourite motivational authors, Wayne Dyer, to turn her mind to a higher meaning. I told her I named her Alexandra Faith for a reason that had become clear. Her name was like her talisman—faith was what she needed to see her through the obstacles in her life. Unlike an object, she could never lose her name. It possessed her wherever she was, available whenever she needed it. I needed it too. Although I didn't share the same struggles in my life, I had lived through a lot of suffering as well. Experiencing Zandra's grief became overwhelming and I needed to keep the faith that we both had a purpose in it. Every day started with hope and ended by turning it over to God when the burden was overwhelming. Although I couldn't say either of us were thriving, I was grateful for her to simply survive.

Just as Zandra was getting into the rhythm of living day to day with her new diagnosis, news came that would strike both of our hearts with grief. Her old friend Ty had died. Ty, which was short for Tyler, was the only friend she had who also had diabetes. The news came flooding in through friends on Snapchat as they all rallied around one another to comprehend the tragic news. The loss of a friend is always heartbreaking, but for Zandra this was crushing. Apparently he had gone to sleep and didn't wake up. That was my worst nightmare, the one that played on my mind when I allowed my fears to get the best of me. As a parent of a diabetic, I knew that this tragedy was real for some parents; however, hearing of it with someone I knew heightened my own fears and brought them closer to the surface of my awareness.

My heart ached with a pain I had never felt before. I deeply hurt for Ty and his parents. They were living every parent's greatest nightmare. I couldn't comprehend their loss nor process it all myself. I couldn't console Zandra and fully realize the loss and the impact it had on me at the same time. The funeral was to be held on Friday, December 8, just two days after what should have been his nineteenth birthday. I wanted to go to the funeral to show support and say a final farewell to Ty. My heart needed to go, to grieve and share whatever love I could with his family and the community who knew and loved him.

I could tell that the church was going to be full. It was a chilly day with a biting wind. The parking lot was so full I had to park a couple of streets away and turn to face the headwind to walk to the church. The chill reminded me of the day I had buried my dad twenty years earlier. Olivia wanted to come to the funeral with me and I was grateful for her presence. I had asked Zandra if she wanted to come, but she insisted that she would be missing too much class time. I knew that the day would be too much for her, yet wondered if she should be there for closure and to feel the support of those who loved Ty. In the end, I trusted her judgment and didn't press her to come, although I was surprised she didn't.

The church was indeed packed. Ty's old hockey team came to remember their friend, all wearing their hockey jerseys. They sat together, forming a support for each other that no doubt touched each person in the room. It was a stark reminder that Ty's was a life gone way too soon. Family and friends continued to fill the church, each silently holding a special relationship they'd had with this young man who was near and dear to their heart. I was reflecting on the last words that I had shared with Ty. It was in my house, although it had been a couple of years previously. He was over with a group of other kids and I asked him how his new pump worked to control his diabetes. I was curious how he managed the transition, as it was just prior to Zandra getting a pump of her own. He smiled, and in a very teen way of expressing his lack of interest in the topic, replied, "Good," followed by a quick smile. I would have loved to talk to him more, but I had learned that no teenager wants to talk about diabetes, so I went back upstairs. His smile could warm the room and I could still feel it. I could see that he had that special connection with everyone who knew him and appreciated that he would talk with Zandra about his own experience from time to time.

The stories that his family shared struck me deeply. They spoke of his love of travel, having recently been to the Philippines with his family. They spoke of his love for his family and friends and his hope to pursue architecture or law. I tried not to imagine what Zandra's life story would look like if it were to play out on a photo collage and in the stories of loved ones. The baby toys displayed in the photos were the same ones we had in our house—all we had to do was swap the child. I started to sob and I couldn't stop. I used every tissue I brought yet it wasn't enough. I cried my heart out, not only for Ty's family, but for all the others who had lost a child, and for my own fear of following in those tragic footprints. I wept like I hadn't in a very long time. I wept long past the service and into the night.

When community comes together to mourn, it helps everyone to heal and to remember. I was grateful for the coming together of our community to help all those who loved Ty to learn to cherish his memory and find the courage to move on. I was frustrated with myself because, although I was part of the community, I didn't know one of our own was struggling. I wondered if there was something I could have done to help. I could imagine myself sitting with Ty, his mom and Zandra, talking about how they have a unique struggle but assuring them they were never alone. I knew he must have been going through some of the same situations that Zandra had and found it equally as difficult. I had often asked Zandra about him. I knew she saw him more than I did. "He's fine, Mom," Zandra would say. When I asked if she wanted to have him over, she replied, "He's got different friends so I don't see him much anymore." Now I wish I'd stayed connected with his mom. I wish I'd supported her through what I know she must have struggled with. She needed to know she wasn't alone, but now she had lost her only child and I still had mine.

In the days following the funeral, my life continued to flow along. I was thankful for the obligations and schedules that help string together time, even when I feel more like a spectator in my life than the main character. Losing Ty was a grave reminder that diabetes can take a precious life away and I never knew what fate had planned in my life. For so long, I had refused to succumb to my own fears. Perhaps this was because I didn't know what to do with them anyhow. There was no use looking at what could happen, so I decided to hold on to hope instead. When Zandra continued to call, feeling hopeless and downtrodden, I fought for hope even harder. I was on a one-woman crusade to pull her out of her agony. I felt I was the only one who could.

The magnitude of the stress had been getting to me. I was exhausted. Everything felt like work and my emotional state threatened to take over the joy in my life. With my three other children, there were so many needs that needed tending to. I felt like diabetes had not only robbed Zandra of her happiness, but mine as well. I decided that I needed a quiet day to myself with a cup of tea and a good book. I had lots of great books to choose from that had been collecting on my nightstand. I knew that not reading regularly was a sign of stress for me. It takes greater energy and imagination to read than to sit in front of the TV, and I had been doing a lot more screen watching. I knew that taking a day was healthy self-care, and I was long overdue.

My mug was steaming and my book cracked open when the phone rang. I knew Zandra was supposed to be in class and wasn't expecting to hear from her. When I looked at my ringing phone, the caller ID confirmed my fears. I knew something was wrong and my heart sank. I tried to offset the pain that I knew was on the other end and answered the phone with the most cheerful hello I could muster. On the other end was despair. In a weak voice, she asked, "Would you be relieved if I died and you didn't have to hear me struggle?" I asked her where she got that idea from. She replied, "In the back of Ty's funeral pamphlet, his family speaks about him being better off with God, that he can finally rest in peace." She asked again, "Would it be better for everyone if I went to be with God?"

Things had been getting worse, but now I had confirmation and alarm bells were going off in my head. I felt panic rising up in my body. I began praying to God to surround her with his angels to console her in this lonely time. I instantly brought forth a vision of angels' wings wrapped around her. I begged for Him to be there when I couldn't. I prayed like a script being played and yet maintained the ability to hold a weak conversation. I told Zandra that when we lose people we love, the only consolation we have is that their earthly suffering is over, because for the one suffering, their physical suffering has ended. I told her that the burden to care for the person is over, but that the pain for those living was certainly not. They could only pray for Ty and turn his care over to God. I told her that nobody wants to hand his or her loved ones over; it isn't by choice. We love fiercely, but so does God. She seemed to understand what I was saying. I told her, "If it were the other way around, and I was struggling and passed away, it wouldn't be because you gave up, but you would take comfort knowing God, who works miracles, was with me." Again, she agreed.

I was making it through the conversation. God was giving me the strength to keep my legs under me and not crumble. I felt as though the words I was speaking were also meant for me. So often this was the case. The strength that I needed in my own life was coming from within myself. I could happily live without having to think of diabetes and the struggles that Zandra was having, but I knew in that moment that I was becoming stronger for it. Now, more than ever, I needed to keep faith that all these struggles were by the design of the hand of God to evolve my soul so I could help others. This was why I had become Alexandra's mom.

CHAPTER 11

Hypnotherapy

"With my mom's genes, you'll live forever," I told Zandra when she called several weeks after the funeral. Ever since Ty's passing, I could tell that things had become more difficult for Zandra. Not only was she struggling to manage school and diabetes, but she was balancing the greater burden of loss and fear. I would often use my mom as an example of strength, albeit not in the most favourable way. My mom has struggled with mental health as far back as I remember. When I was a teenager, I found out that she was bulimic after Karen had blurted it out in one of our many teenage scraps. I was shocked. It was the first time I had external confirmation that something was wrong with Mom. Everything up to that point had been based on Mom's disclosure or my own observations. It wasn't uncommon to watch Mom inhale a full loaf of bread and the best part of a pound of butter in the morning with her coffee and newspaper, but I had accepted these types of indulgences as something familiar and didn't question them. I assumed she kept her petite figure because she had genes that were not passed down to me. I accepted her binges as normal, as a part of her quirkiness.

Mom also suffered from a severe addiction to prescription drugs. Normal morning sounds were Mom rising from bed, heading to the bathroom to use the toilet, then the predictable shuffling of pills in a bottle. A sure way to know Mom was up was to hear the medicine cabinet and the rattling of her pills. When I was little and wanted to be like Mom, I would keep my old rocket candies from Halloween in a discarded pill bottle in my bathroom and shake one or two out every day before I left the bathroom. My desire to connect with my mom and follow in her footsteps allowed me to mimic even the worst of her habits. I never realized that she had an addiction until I was in Grade 9. Once the door was opened and I began to see the struggles she was dealing with, the final shreds of my naive and trusting youth were severed. It was as if in a matter of weeks the rug had been pulled out from under me and I didn't understand the world that I was living in. I wanted to turn the page and end the chapter where the suspense was heightened. I wanted out of my life and the pain that was inescapable. Everything I thought I knew about myself and my family was unfamiliar, and inside I felt despondent.

With a new lens, I could see the unhealthy patterns and addictions that were hiding in plain sight for so long. I realized that Mom was stoned most of the time, so often that at times she couldn't drive home from the store. Throughout her life, she had consumed so many prescription drugs that she began to look like a junkie. I confronted her in my best effort to help and support her. I was desperate to make up for what she was lacking in her life and genuinely felt that I could be the difference between her destructive lifestyle and the one she deserved. After my pleas with her, it seemed as though she no longer felt the need to put any effort into covering up her lifestyle.

When I was about ten, my mom was diagnosed with rheumatoid arthritis, the same diagnosis as her mom. As the disease progressed, her joints became visibly gnarled and twisted, not to mention intensely painful. Mom has struggled with dangerously high blood pressure, bowel trouble and mental health for as long as I can remember. Our family has been told countless times that she wouldn't live much longer, yet she somehow has defied the odds and is still living, and she is now in her seventies. Although she's not the picture of health, she's likely to live another decade or more, so I figure with those genes the rest of her family by default has got to be tough. More times than I can count the family has been told she won't live through the night because of her dangerously high blood pressure, but she's pulled through to the surprise of even the most experienced medical professionals.

Reminding Zandra of her Nanna always lightens the mood. It wouldn't be so funny if it wasn't for the lightness with which Mom looks upon her lifestyle herself. "If I haven't killed myself by my own actions, nothing will!" she has said. "We have strong genes in our family—built like ox," she muses whenever she can. Retelling this to Zandra takes the intense spotlight off her own troubles and diffuses it with humour, because she understands the truth. People can and have lived through incredible disease and come out the other end to live long, happy and triumphant lives. Although it would be a stretch to call my mom "triumphant," she does seem to bumble along, seemingly careless about the outcome of her next health crisis.

I have always had open conversations about my mom with the kids. I like to tell them stories about both my parents that place them in the best light, acknowledging that they are people who did the best they could with what they had. I try to teach them to have forgiving hearts, because when people know better, they do better. Sometimes we automatically do exactly what we learn. This mindset has helped me to forgive both my parents for the emotional abuse and neglect that I experienced growing up. Now I can change their legacies by focusing on those things they did that were good and loving, and that demonstrated the best of them. This narrative has not only refocused my attention, but has also changed history by bringing truth and light to mental illness. I have found a new way to honour my mother and my father by choosing to see and tell the story of the best of them.

By honouring them, I like to point out how much Joseph is like his grandfather. He not only looks just like him, but he has the same kind, loving soul as my dad. I like to tell Olivia that she has the green thumb of her Nanna as well as her sharp wit. Liam has the same sharp wit, but with the same looks that came down from Nanna. He has my grandfather's dimples and mischievous smile. Zandra has Mom's olive skin and determination. These are all amazing qualities and gifts passed down from their grandparents. Recognizing these qualities that I love in my children is how I honour my parents. I grieve for the two-way, loving relationship that I have never had with Mom. Whenever I realize that my thoughts are falling into the old mental tape-recording of loss and grief, I send her love and focus on the gifts I have because of her.

During this time in my life I learned how to capture moments that gave me peace. If I could make someone smile, I captured that feeling and held on to it like a freshly picked flower on a walk. I could never guarantee what the next moment brought, so I chose to live in the present. I have watched moms who love to worry. I've never desired to be one of them. I heard once that worry is like saying a prayer for the very thing you don't want. I've heard Wayne Dyer say, "Where attention goes, energy flows" so many times. I choose to look to the outcome I want and then deal with what was meant to be in the end. But I've been tested.

Despite coming from strong stock, Zandra felt weak and afraid from her physical struggles. She was finding herself getting up in the night to test her blood sugars and, when she tested low, overdoing the corresponding snack. This was causing extremely high blood sugars in the morning that were increasing her overall A1C. This pattern started off small, overdoing a correction here and there, but quickly snowballed again into waking up every night to eat. The habit quickly turned into something she struggled to manage. It grew like an addiction, and, like an addict, she hid it from the rest of the world. She never told me about it in the beginning, but I noticed the hostile and angry feelings she had toward herself. I noticed them in how she shamed her body for not looking as she did in Grade 12 and for the gruelling exercise regimen she felt she needed to keep. It wasn't the kind of exercise that came about through loving one's self, more the kind that punished it.

Zandra finally broke down and told me, "I've been watching TV and eating before bed so I don't wake up low." I immediately knew she was scared to die in her sleep like her friend Ty had. "This is fear, honey," I assured her. "This is something we can deal with." I could completely understand her fear; however, I didn't know how to help her. Despite having opened up about what she was doing, she continued eating at night and waking with dangerously high blood sugar in the morning. The more this pattern continued, the worse the self-hatred and loathing grew.

I suggested we crack the pattern by letting someone know when it was happening. We decided together that she would call me when she had snacked too much before bed, or during the night. Creating this plan allowed me some peace in an otherwise deeply disturbing time.

We both felt confident that this would help. I would make sure to check in before bed with a quick text to assure her she was on my mind. We would exchange loving emoticons that settled my mind before bed, only to do another check-in in the morning to find out she snacked again and had a blood sugar three or four times what it should have been.

Zandra's fear had gone too far. I felt as if she was in crisis again. A couple of years prior I had taken courses and completed my practicum to become a certified hypnotherapist. I had been having severe migraines caused by the pain in my jaw for some time and it was getting much worse. One night, I was halfway home from Edmonton and a migraine hit. I had to pull over, and luckily I had some painkillers in my purse. I had to wait until they kicked in before I could continue to drive home. These kinds of headaches were becoming normal and the clicking in my jaw was showing wear in my TM joint—the hinge between jawbone and skull—in my most recent dental X-rays. A friend of mine had suggested that I see a hypnotherapist when all other avenues to help with my pain were failing, but at the time I didn't see how it would help. I reached the point that I would do anything to make the pain stop, so I called Padman Pillai, the hypnotherapist she had seen so long ago. I was glad to see that he was still in business. I met with this little spritely man of East Indian descent. He was in his eighties, but you wouldn't know it. The appointment lasted three hours, but we spent the first hour building a rapport and understanding what I needed. He told me he had helped numerous clients with TMJ pain and that it was actually quite common, as we often hold trauma in the jaw. I didn't feel as though I could be hypnotized, but I decided to trust his process and he assured me that he had a lot of tools in his toolbox for difficult clients.

The experience was quite interesting—relaxing, to say the least. I decided to give it another week to see if I needed to go back for a follow-up. I didn't have a single headache that week! I hadn't gone that long without a headache or jaw pain for a long time. I still had a ringing in my ear and decided to go back. The second appointment was easier: I knew what to expect and trusted the process. He told me that the pain may return, but I could heal it myself and he showed me how to hold my hand on my jaw and bring healing energy to it. I didn't believe that it would be gone because I had lived with it for so long, starting with an episode of lockjaw when I was a teenager, but I had felt much better that week, which encouraged me to keep going. After several months without painful headaches or jaw pain, I knew I needed to learn the process. I needed to know what he did so that I could help bring healing to those I care about. I looked up Padman's website and saw that he was a teacher and had an upcoming class. The process wasn't cheap and would take several months of classes, followed up by a practicum, but I was determined.

During my training I learned that hypnosis was used in everyday advertising, and that we take suggestions from nearly everything around us. These suggestions become how we view ourselves and can become very unhelpful, causing a lot of disruption in our lives. Our beliefs are shaped from messages in our environment and can be unhealthy for us if we're hearing the wrong ones. Hypnotherapy can work as a way to reset our beliefs to a healthy state. When a person experiences a traumatic event, they can develop a belief that they're not valuable, or are unworthy. Sometimes we develop a confirmation of fear, which becomes a phobia, or we believe that we're not worthy of love, even though we can recognize that all the factors around us tell us this isn't true. The subconscious remembers the event, and when a belief is deep in the subconscious, we act out our beliefs even though it's not what we want. Hypnotherapy works by directly accessing the subconscious and altering the message to one that serves the person in a healthy way. The very first client I had in my practicum had been a smoker for over twenty-five years. He wanted to quit smoking and chewing tobacco. After just one session, he gave up his belief that he needed to smoke to be cool. He was ready for the change and just needed help to change his mindset.

It was time I used my training on Zandra. I knew I could help her with her fear, but I also knew that my connection to her as a parent could either strengthen the experience or impair it. I had to at least try. I asked her if she was willing to work with me when she came home on the weekend, and to my surprise she was. She clearly wanted to resolve this fear that held her hostage as well. That Friday, her red Ford Focus rolled up with Cinnamon in the back seat excited to be home as well. We planned to do the hypnotherapy session the following morning so we could have a quiet house. We didn't have to worry about the Friday night, because when she was home she felt safe and didn't need to overeat in the night.

"Close your eyes and allow your body to relax where it is, with your arms loose at your sides and your legs uncrossed," I started. It wasn't long before she was in a deep trance. I had prepared for our session with a focus greater than any other I had before. I had my scripts tailored to her needs and had walked her through the process, so she knew what to expect. When I had finished, I counted down and she didn't want to open her eyes. I tried again and again, without any luck. I could ask her to raise her hand and she immediately complied, yet she wouldn't open her eyes. I was trained for this. My instructor had taught us that some people are enjoying such a pleasant state without worry and stress that their subconscious doesn't want to end it. I was taught how to navigate this scenario, so I wasn't worried. Experiencing this with Zandra only proved to me how she needed the welcome escape from her reality. She felt safe, knowing she was watched and that nothing bad would happen. For me, it was already a success. I gave her this rest, this comfort, and all my training was worth it in that moment.

When she opened her eyes, she described being in a beautiful forest that she didn't want to leave. She felt safe and very relaxed, more relaxed than she had been in a long, long time. Time would tell how the suggestions in our session would impact her life. I had learned in my training that, although we want the best for our clients, to solve all their problems and turn their lives around for the better, we have to be unattached to that outcome. Our egos want us to be the ones who solve people's problems, to be the ones who knew what to do and receive the accolades, but we are only instruments of healing, not the healing source. Sometimes we can see the major shifts within days, and sometimes the shift that eventually gives way to the bigger change is etching away under the surface, unseen by anyone. I was happy to be able to give Zandra the comfort I know she needed and let her and God determine what needed to be done.

When Zandra went back to Edmonton on Sunday night, she was feeling great. She was sad to leave home but had felt really good while she was back in the family nest. Unfortunately, the snacking resumed after a stressful day at school near the beginning of the week, resulting in sky-high blood sugar levels and even more inward shame. I realized at the time that we had only scratched the surface with our first hypnotherapy session, and that the root of the problem was going to take some time. As her mother, giving up wasn't an option. Helping Zandra find her way was my purpose and nobody could do it as well as I could. I had often felt a deep sense of hurt and self-pity at her age, yet growing up I didn't have someone who could support me. Lord knows I needed it. This was my new purpose, a way to right the wrongs and protect the future generation from the roadblocks that I had stumbled on for so long in my life.

Inside I knew that Zandra's binge eating came from me. As a child, I was known in my family as the skinny one. I naturally loved to be active and didn't have much appetite. I had a take-it-or-leave-it attitude with food, never feeling the compulsion to overeat or take what I didn't want, even if it was something as tempting as chocolate. This predisposition was helpful in a house that imparted that people who are overweight were unlovable. As I got older and began noticing my mom's habits of binge eating, I somehow took overeating on sweets as my own coping method, without the aftereffect of purging. Over time, this resulted in a steady weight gain throughout my adult life. Although I would consider my diet to be healthy, consisting of fruits and vegetables and limited sources of artificial colours, flavours and preservatives, in times of stress I headed to the chocolate and indulged without limits. If I could take on this way of coping from my mom, surely Zandra could as well. Combined with her need to control her sugars to survive and her fear of not waking up, this factor coalesced into one big, complicated problem that would take time to sort through.

Hypnotherapy was proving to be useful even if we weren't ready to reach the goal we had set out toward. During the nights, when Zandra would test low, she found it hard to limit her low treatment to a reasonable amount of carbs, or sugar. The usual protocol for a low is to treat it with fifteen grams of sugar carbs and wait fifteen minutes before you retest. If you're still low, you have another fifteen grams of carbs and include a carbohydrate snack to raise the blood sugar and hold it until morning, or the next meal. Zandra was having a hard time waiting the fifteen minutes. Instead, she would start panicking that she needed more, giving in to the shaky, unstable feeling of low blood sugar. I created a recording that lasted fifteen minutes that she could use to fill the time while she waited. This recording included many of the aspects of hypnotherapy without deepening them. The recording was intended to be calming and reassuring, to remind her that her body was always working on her behalf and functioned on the same intelligence that beat her heart, breathed air into her lungs and grew her hair. I assured her that her body knows exactly what to do and she didn't have to be in full control in that moment. This recording became so helpful that she used it every night, and its message eventually took hold.

I created another recording for her to listen to as she went into sleep, assuring her that her body would let her know if she needed to wake up because of low blood sugar, allowing her a peaceful and restful sleep in the meanwhile. The key for Zandra was giving her permission to let go and not be in full control in every minute. The need for control for a diabetic is understandable, although takes its toll emotionally and becomes exhausting.

Yet another recording was created after a stressed phone conversation we had one morning. Zandra had another statistics class that was even harder than the first. She was feeling overwhelmed and assured me that she didn't know a lot of what she was reviewing, and the test was in the afternoon. "How can I review material and do well on a test when what I'm reviewing is new material?" Zandra was completely overwhelmed. She always tried her best, but when it came to statistics, she didn't seem to retain what she read. Her anxiety wasn't from lack of trying, but from not believing that she could do well. Her pattern of stressful and sleepless nights didn't help matters either. I felt at a loss as to what I could suggest, but experience has taught me that panic studying only serves to enhance the stress of the situation. I told her that I would create a recording and send it right to her. I told her to stop studying and listen to the recording a couple times before the exam. She agreed to do what I suggested.

I promptly pulled a couple of scripts that I like to use for relaxing and knew I only had time to ad lib the rest. I sat on my office floor, played some relaxing music in the background and set my iPhone to record. I created a recording that I hoped would take her out of her stressed state by encouraging her to notice certain feelings in her physical body, then suggesting that she feel assured that the material that she does know is solidly memorized and able to be recalled on her exam with ease. A lot of understanding goes into the language used to help someone accept the suggestions, and I used all of my resources to create an effective recording. When I sent the recording to her, I said a prayer that my suggestions for her were able to help, along with a prayer of gratitude that I could offer something, even a simple recording, to demonstrate my love and concern for her.

"I can't believe it, I passed!" Zandra called to tell me a couple of days later. She described feeling calm during her exam and being able to recall all of the material she knew, focusing on that rather than what she wasn't as confident in. Slowly, very slowly, I felt as if we were chipping away at the hard shell that housed the vulnerability in Zandra that she needed to expose and heal. I felt an inner knowledge that these lessons were by design, to teach us both what we needed in our lives. I could feel that Zandra had an unforgiving heart, mostly toward herself, that prevented her from fully expressing love. For me, I felt as though the shame and pain that sat dormant in the dark recesses of my being were slowly being called out. I couldn't name it, yet I felt I had a purpose, as if my own trauma was the prerequisite for the understanding I needed now. To understand pain is to have felt it. To help someone find their way through it I needed to have explored it fully myself, co-existing with shame until it overstayed its welcome and was finally cast away.

The encouragement I felt from knowing I helped Zandra over another hurdle reinforced my belief that I was on the right path. I felt a sense of purpose knowing that I was of use in this situation, and I could see the proof that what limits us lies within the constraints of our own mind. The victory in my heart wasn't one I could shout from the rooftops, yet it was one that gave me some confidence. I used this belief to encourage myself in my own abilities to help others, as well as to bolster faith in myself that I already possessed what I needed to be of service. I may not know stats, but I can help those who do to feel confident in what they know, at least enough to pass the course.

CHAPTER 12

A Fearful Heart

FEAR CAN MASK ITSELF IN many ways and implant itself in any situation. Zandra was exceptionally hard on herself, for not only her diabetes, but for negative behaviours like watching Netflix and eating, which occurred when she was in high stress. She hadn't yet fully grieved and healed from her diabetes and thyroid diagnosis, much less processed her feelings and emotions from them. She described feeling betrayed by her own body. Self-betrayal is worse than being betrayed by another, as the anger is then pointed inward and has nowhere else to go. It makes that person their very own villain. I also suspected that long-held traumas from her dad and me divorcing and my remarrying and having another child held deep grief that had never been healed as well.

The tumultuous feelings Zandra was experiencing came in crashing waves that pummelled her without allowing her time to catch her breath before the next one knocked her down. She felt exhausted, and so did I. The exhaustion and negative feelings became like drugs she used to soothe herself when she was hurting. It became a cycle that often spiralled out of control and became a distraction from the intensity of the emotion rooted beneath it. She felt alone and ashamed, and she was becoming withdrawn. She needed a break, a physical emancipation from her diseased body, but realized that no such respite existed. No matter how much I wanted and was willing to help, she had to find her own way, we all do. Seeing her suffer changed me. I've heard it said that a mother is only as happy as her unhappiest child, and I knew this all too well. No matter how much fun I appeared to be having, a part of my heart was aching. A part of me was always with Zandra, feeling the pain she was in. I tried to settle the distress signals by sending beacons of love and light to her, having faith that they would be received, although I would never be able to measure the difference.

After Christmas, when the break was over and school was gearing up, I got the feeling things were getting worse, despite the strides we had made with hypnotherapy. When I would talk to Zandra on the phone, she was often running in the river valley. She always loved the outdoors and the valley trails were beautiful, yet she wasn't on them for the beauty. She was running to offset her high blood sugars from eating too much and the negative body image she was forming.

When Zandra was around twelve, one of her favourite things to do in the spring was play soccer. She had proven herself to be a valuable defensive player and eventually took over the position of keeper. She helped bring many victories to her league and built confidence in herself as an athlete. Goalies get a lot of bruises. Zandra would often come home from a game and treat her scrapes and sores. She was always covered in bruises on her shins, which became very sore. Because she went from soccer to volleyball to all manner of outdoor sports, including riding horses, the bruises never seemed to heal. From time to time she would inquire about them at the doctor's office, but because she was so active it was easy to pass them off as sports related. Eventually her shins grew worse, even after she quit soccer in high school. Her shins would ache and slow her down on runs. Both of us tried tirelessly to figure out what it could be, but the closest we could find, although it was a stretch, was that it was shin splints. The answer was for her to take a break from running, which didn't feel to her like an answer at all. Despite all the doctor's warnings not to use exercise to manage daily blood sugars—to use it to manage long-term health only—she constantly did so. She would continually go for a workout or a run to bring down high blood sugars. She felt as if the higher the amount of insulin needed, the worse a diabetic she was, so she tried to achieve a lower number by planning an activity with each meal. She felt shame needing to use more insulin, and although I would call her out on it she never changed her behaviour. Now, these runs were causing great pain to her legs.

When I would talk to Zandra on the phone, she often spoke about the pain in her legs. When I would see her, I was able to see how the bruising was getting wider and redder. I would suggest to her that she should take a break, which only upset and angered her. She became insolent and continued to press on running. She continued to run as a punishment to her body for having diabetes and thyroid disease. The cycle of fear, anger and punishment pushed her to run harder, a daily retribution to her emotional state. These calls during her runs were often filled with sobs of despair, and they eventually created fear and panic in her most loved companion, Cinnamon.

"Cinnamon pooped at school with her vest on!" Zandra said in a panicked call. Although I knew it was always wrong for a dog to poop with a vest on, the image that came to mind was funny to me. I started laughing while I imagined sweet Cinnamon walking along the sidewalk in her red vest, with her uptight handler speed-walking to class. Although I knew it was humiliating for her, I couldn't help but find the humour. Cinnamon is a well-behaved dog, but as I reminded Zandra, she's a living and breathing animal that can at times be unpredictable. I wasn't exactly sure why she called me, but I quickly caught on that she needed a distraction. She needed to vent. She became angry with Cinnamon, which hurt and upset me. She had been complaining about how Cinnamon was slow and holding her back during runs. She had even complained just days before that Cinnamon wasn't listening properly when out on a walk the week before. "She just sits there and shakes," Zandra told me weeks later when Cinnamon had another episode of not listening.

Cinnamon was checked out at the vet and released with a clean bill of health. There was nothing wrong with her physically, yet the complaints continued. Zandra called me on her way to school one morning: "She is refusing to walk," she exclaimed. "I don't want to take her anymore!" I thought we had moved past these issues. I hardly had energy to keep up with the new stresses, much less go back and repeat old ones. My frustration was increasing and I was having a hard time managing her frequent distress calls, yet I was fearful of cutting them off. The vet had indicated that Cinnamon was starting to get arthritis in her hips, although it wasn't significant yet, or at the level where it needed to be managed by medication. It seemed strange to me that Cinnamon was acting up, yet I wasn't putting a lot of mental energy into it either. I had a lot going on in my own life, managing all the aspects of a family with three other children. I had hoped that Zandra being in the second semester, having passed the first round of exams, would have allowed some settling, resulting in more pleasant exchanges.

"I'm so angry with her," Zandra cried. "She's such a bad dog and I can't deal with it anymore." She had told me that she was acting like this every time she went out on a walk. Suddenly it clicked. I knew what was going on. "Is she okay when you're not on the phone?" I asked, feeling confident I knew the answer.

"I'm not sure," she said.

"You often call me while walking her when you're not feeling your best," I said, trying to soften the blow. "When you talk to Devin, are you out running or walking as well, and are you also upset?"

"Well, yes," she responded.

"Cinnamon has PTSD," I replied. I felt sure of it. If I was feeling stressed and I was only on the phone for twenty minutes at a time with her, surely Cinnamon was even more distressed than me. If Zandra was on the phone crying and feeling heightened emotion, Cinnamon would feel like the phone was something bad and upsetting to her.

It all made sense, and the more I thought it through, the clearer the writing was on the wall. Once I made the connection, I felt as if I could tap into Cinnamon and all of the confirmation I needed came through. The last time I saw her, she looked nervous: her eyes were darting, and she was even clingier to Zandra than usual. Perhaps I felt I could relate to the stress she was experiencing. The good news was that there was a way to help her through it, but it meant Zandra would have to acknowledge and change things.

Once I explained things to Zandra, she quickly realized that what I was saying made sense. She tested the theory out on her next walk. She went out, and after a while she called me. "She's doing it," she said. "As soon as I picked up my phone and started talking, she started eye-darting and looking stressed." She felt enormous despair as she realized that her actions were so far-reaching that they had impacted Cinnamon in this way. This new revelation was hopeful yet disheartening. The burden of causing someone else to suffer was distressing, yet knowing that she could also be the source of healing gave hope and light to a dark time.

Zandra realized that she needed to connect to Cinnamon without outside sources at play. When they went on walks, it was back to basics—for the joy of getting out. When Cinnamon was off leash, jumping up and over tree stumps, something Zandra named "lopping"—short for log hopping—it was just the two of them at play, no phones allowed. This intended play was cathartic for both Zandra and Cinnamon, and it created the foundation of permission that she needed to let go and have fun. It worked. Before long, Cinnamon was playfully walking along trails and following Zandra to class. Any time Zandra would return to her old ways, allowing her frustrations to spill over into her walks, Cinnamon would revert to her familiar distress; and provided Zandra the immediate feedback needed to correct her ways.

When winter turned into spring and final exams were behind her, Zandra decided to leave the condo and come home for the summer. This decision was frustrating to us. Bills still had to be paid, and now we were supporting two households, but after experiencing such a difficult year we knew she needed to be home amongst the busyness of our bustling family and activities. She bolstered her decision by offering to help with the errands and driving her brothers to their activities. She was also able to pick shifts up at Lammles, the Western-wear store she had been working at for a couple of years. Lammles had always supported Zandra's diabetic needs and encouraged Cinnamon to be with her at work, even providing her with her own name tag.

At the end of May, I planned a trip with Karen and Zandra to fly to Victoria. We would spend some time on Vancouver Island and drive to Tofino in a rented car. I knew that Zandra had had a difficult year and I secretly wanted to impress upon her the benefits of a fresh start. I thought that the Island would do her good—forests were always healing for me and I thought that they could be for her as well. Visiting Victoria with her would be a perk for me too.

The trip was amazing. I had been to Vancouver Island for the first time a couple of years prior with Gord, when we had come as a couple on a very belated honeymoon. We both instantly fell in love with it and knew that somehow we would end up residents, even if only in retirement. We drove along the highway, shaded by the ancient cedar trees, with both the ocean and the mountains in view. It was breathtaking and I was surprised that such beauty was only a province away. I wanted Zandra to know that she could live in this magic if she decided to.

Upon landing at the Nanaimo airport, Zandra expressed that the air pressure had caused a burst in her mouth. She'd had her wisdom teeth removed a week earlier and now felt as if something was infected. The day before we left, she checked in with our dentist, Dr. Dinh. She wasn't having a lot of pain, but her intuition told her something wasn't quite right. Although everything checked out okay, Dr. Dinh prescribed Zandra an antibiotic just in case an infection appeared while we were gone. She made sure to fill the prescription and have it on hand. After what felt like a burst of an infection in her mouth, Zandra decided to start taking the antibiotics right away. We left the airport and secured our rental car, and she rummaged through her bag for her antibiotics. It wasn't long before we were on the highway, speeding our way toward Tofino.

We spent a lot of time on the balcony, enjoying wine, brie and crackers while watching the bald eagles soaring right over our heads. We were in full view of the seaplanes taking off and could watch the pilots fuel and prepare their planes for passengers.

On our first morning in Tofino, Zandra came upstairs to the bedroom that opened to large windows, which took advantage of the expansive views of the waterway. She asked me to check out her mouth. She had lightly touched her cheek and felt a burst, followed by a foul taste. It was clear she had an infection, and whenever her body was fighting something her blood sugars rose high. We had found the answer, but now needed help. We called Dr. Dinh, who had graciously included his cell number on his card. We hoped that he would answer on a Sunday morning. He did, and carefully listened to Zandra describe what had happened. He agreed that it seemed to be an infection, although he was working with us remotely, which made the diagnosis even harder. I was concerned about the infection entering her bloodstream, and so was he. He was also concerned for diabetes complications. Zandra's blood sugars were much higher than normal. She was reluctant to share her blood sugars with him when he asked. We had become accustomed to seeing the highs since we had set out on the trip; however, we pressed on and didn't pay it as much attention as we perhaps should have. His inquiry snapped me back into reality, reminding me that there are no days off from being diabetic. Dr. Dinh explained that antibiotics tend to increase blood sugar and had no blame or disrespect for what she was experiencing. These factors combined with the infection could be what was driving her increased blood sugars. He expressed that he would have his phone all day and evening should we have any further concerns. He advised that Zandra continue to take her antibiotics and urged us to visit a clinic or hospital if her symptoms got worse. His care and concern appeased my fears, knowing that there were always helpers when we needed them.

Tofino was spectacular. We toured the area by kayak and watched sea otters and starfish amongst the rocks. We took hikes through the rainforest, walking along the boardwalks that wound around thousand-year-old cedars. On our last day, we drove back to Victoria to visit my Great-Aunty Dolly and Uncle Roy from my dad's side. They had moved to the Island from Calgary over twenty years before. They treated us to a beautiful meal at their favourite restaurant, the Beach House, where we had an ocean-view table and I enjoyed the best mushroom risotto I have ever had. After Uncle Roy heard that we were hoping Zandra would consider going to the University of Victoria, they took us for a drive to see the campus. It looked to me like a little village built around a large circle, with enormous trees and running trails meandering through the campus buildings. Although our visit was short, Zandra had seen enough: she decided to apply to the University of Victoria once we returned home. The university didn't offer the same program she was enrolled in at the University of Alberta, but that didn't matter to her. She was disillusioned with that program after learning in one class that the effects of certain foods and preservatives do harm to the cells in a human body, yet in another class she was told that they ought not share that information with patients, as the government has approved it in specific quantities. To Zandra, it was one or the other. Although cases could be made regarding how preservatives allow greater food distribution and increase shelf life, she refused to support any notion that it was acceptable to eat these poisons, no matter what the government allowed. After a few weeks, she received her acceptance in the biology program at the University of Victoria.

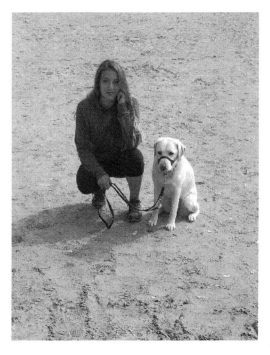

Zandra and Cinnamon on a beach in Tofino

CHAPTER 13

The Big Move

Excitement was in the air. Zandra was moving toward the fresh start that she deserved. She was full of nervous energy as she began to plan her classes and watch the virtual tours online. Together we mapped out the areas around campus that she would like to visit and would need access to, such as groceries and pet stores. Planning for the future became a welcome activity and signalled, to me, the end of many of the stresses from the past. In my heart, I felt that the warmer temperatures, green forests and smaller campus would help steady the course of her wandering vessel toward a brighter horizon.

We didn't know any other students, so I felt it best we look to dorms as the best type of housing. She applied and was denied. The campus housing department explained that first-year students were given a priority for housing and that there weren't any additional rooms available. We were upset, but not crestfallen. There had to be another way. Gord called the university and spoke with someone who was responsible for housing delegation. He explained the situation, including her hypoglycaemic unawareness and her resultant need to be closer to campus. The person he spoke with suggested that we include the details of her condition and specific need for close accommodation and resubmit the application. When Zandra sent the original application, she had included that she was diabetic and had a service dog, but for her to be accepted they needed to know how this set her apart from other residents with disabilities.

Zandra felt unworthy of a dorm room. She explained that taking a room could mean keeping it from a person who was more needy, something she felt uncomfortable with. It took a while for her to accept our position and acknowledge our fears of her living alone. She was a special case and needed to be supported. The new application was submitted and we received housing approval just a couple of weeks before school started.

I had a trip planned of my own. After a lifetime of dreaming about going to Africa, it was finally coming to fruition. I had signed up with Wild Women Expeditions for a photo safari trip to Tanzania, Africa. I had asked several friends if they wanted to join me, but the timing wasn't right for anyone. In the end, I realized that if I wanted to go, I was going solo. I wanted to experience the wonders of Africa with other women, and for my own safety I wanted to belong to a group, so when Gord mentioned that he had been seeing posts from Wild Women Expeditions, it just felt right. I signed up in the beginning of January 2018 and spent the next nine months preparing for one of the best adventures of my life. When I signed up, I chose to arrive several days ahead of the group. I wanted to spend some time resting and touring the city of Arusha. Since the group was meeting at a hotel not far from the Kilimanjaro airport, I knew that I could easily stay a few days on my own and hire a taxi to take me around. My flight left on September 5, which meant I wouldn't be around for the first or second week of school. I had planned to fly with Zandra to Victoria, but my trip was going to have to be short. I had less than twenty-four hours to get her settled and return home before I headed to Africa.

When we arrived in Victoria, we had to hustle. We had to attend the orientation and get Zandra set up with her key and laundry card, as well as find the bookstore and get her the essentials for her room, all in less than a full day. We stayed at a cheap hotel and headed out for some shopping on the first night. We came across the most glamorous big-box store we had ever seen, with underground parking and elevators to the second floor! We looked at the stack of refrigerators and determined that we wanted a smaller size. We went about buying towels, soaps, pillows, a broom and all the other necessities that we hadn't brought from home. We decided to look around town for a smaller fridge, so we went to several other stores, but could not find any. We decided to settle on the larger fridge from the store we had first attended, but when we returned they were all sold out. I couldn't believe it—they'd had dozens only a few hours earlier! We left empty-handed and upset: Zandra would need a fridge in which to keep her insulin.

The next morning was campus orientation. We packed our suitcases and checked out of the hotel. We were headed for campus, where I would get her settled in, and I had to leave by early afternoon to return home. The parking lot was full yet organized, as second- and third-year students held signs ushering us to a spot to park. We had no idea where to go, but quickly found the lineup of other excited students who were queuing up for their room keys. The campus had an amazing energy. Tables and tents were set up, each one welcoming the newbies and their families and highlighting the events happening in the year. There was music playing on the loudspeakers, keeping the vibe upbeat and cheery. Even the weather was cooperating. It was a truly gorgeous day on the Island with a warm sun and a cool ocean breeze. I was excited. I had never experienced the dorm life for myself. I graduated from the Northern Alberta Institute of Technology, where on-site student living wasn't an option, so I lived in a small one-bedroom apartment nearby.

This experience was new to me and not at all what I expected. I loved it. I felt like Deanne, the middle-aged mother played by Melissa McCarthy in the movie *Life of the Party*. I wanted to stay and enjoy the fun. I could see myself as a student in that moment. I didn't have the fears that I held in my teenage years and I knew that I was a much better version of my younger self. I had held on to an emptiness for years of what could have been. Several of my friends talked about their university days with such joy. They would reminisce about the old days when they would go to the bars then cram for exams. My life at the time was filled with loss and grief. I allowed the fun of my college years to pass me by, but given a second chance I could see how different the experience would be.

I could see the fear in Zandra's eyes as she clutched Cinnamon's leash and walked from table to table with me. I knew and understood her fear, yet also knew she would grow out of it, just like I had. I still have fears, only different ones. The realization of this became a marker of growth that I silently celebrated. I needed all the encouragement I could give myself, as my fears of travelling alone to Africa had begun to build. Soon it would be my turn to be left alone in a strange place.

In one of the buildings on campus, we could see refrigerators being sold. They were double the cost of the ones at Walmart, but I was prepared to buy one out of necessity. Once we were handed the room key, we went back out to the car and hauled out all her belongings. We were overloaded with move-in necessities, the same as any other new student. It was such a funny scene, all those kids and their parents with bundles piled high, that I took a photo. It was a special moment, as well as humorous. On the outside of each door, the names of the new tenants were written in sharpie on cut-out construction paper. Each one served as a welcome and an opportunity to meet the neighbours. This small gesture was touching. I could see the spirit of the campus, and as I walked along I was curious who her neighbours were.

The rooms were tiny. Each held a single bed, wardrobe and small desk. There wasn't a lot of room to walk around but enough to hold everything she would need. Over the next hour, we busied ourselves with making up the beds with sheets in her favourite shade of yellow, setting up her binders, and hanging her clothes. We had even bought a big bag of dog food and made up a place for Cinnamon by the main-floor window. Once we were sufficiently unpacked and settled, we decided to figure out where the laundry facilities were, purchase a fridge, and, if we had time, look around the campus a little more.

On our way out of her dorm room, we met her new neighbour, Lucy, who was also with her mom. Lucy was a first-year psychology student from Vancouver. She was kind and outgoing. As we stood in the hall, both moms and girls chatting and going through introductions, Lucy quickly offered Zandra her fridge when she heard that we were headed out to buy one. She had already bought one and, as neighbours, was willing to share until Zandra found her own. Zandra was frugal, and even though I was offering to purchase the fridge, she insisted that she would find one cheaper on Craigslist. I wanted to press, but at the same time wanted Zandra to foster a friendship with her new neighbour, so I let it be.

Once we were back outside, we decided to walk around the campus and look at the science buildings that she would likely attend classes in. The vegetation was tall, lush and still flowering, quite a contrast to our Alberta varieties. We enjoyed seeing the green spaces with the traditional totem poles on display in them. We even found a gated trail that held several labelled varieties of plant species, safe away from the high deer population, known as Finnerty Gardens. The path was so peaceful, one that I knew would become a quick favourite for Zandra and Cinnamon.

After what felt like a rushed trip, my time had come to an end. I had to leave for the airport. As we made our way back to the car, the air felt uncomfortably heavy. We'd had so much fun up to this point. Now was the time to truly let her fly out of the nest. I knew that I was her lifeline and that I would be out of contact with her for at least a couple weeks. As much as I didn't want to leave, I knew that it was meant to be. As we walked closer to the car, I could hear Zandra's emotions becoming harder to control. She was terrified. I could tell that her fear was less about the unknown and more about the returning sadness that she knew all too well. As much as I wanted to take over, I knew that she needed to find her way without me. She needed to dig deep, past her pain, to find her strength. I knew that once she did, she would grow to become what she was meant to be. I needed to encourage and not enable. She needed to know how far she could soar. In many ways, she had already outgrown me. She had already moved out of our province, something I never did. She had already proved her academic success to earn her a place in a second university, something I had self-sabotaged for myself. As I drove to the airport, tears of pride fell heavily on my lap.

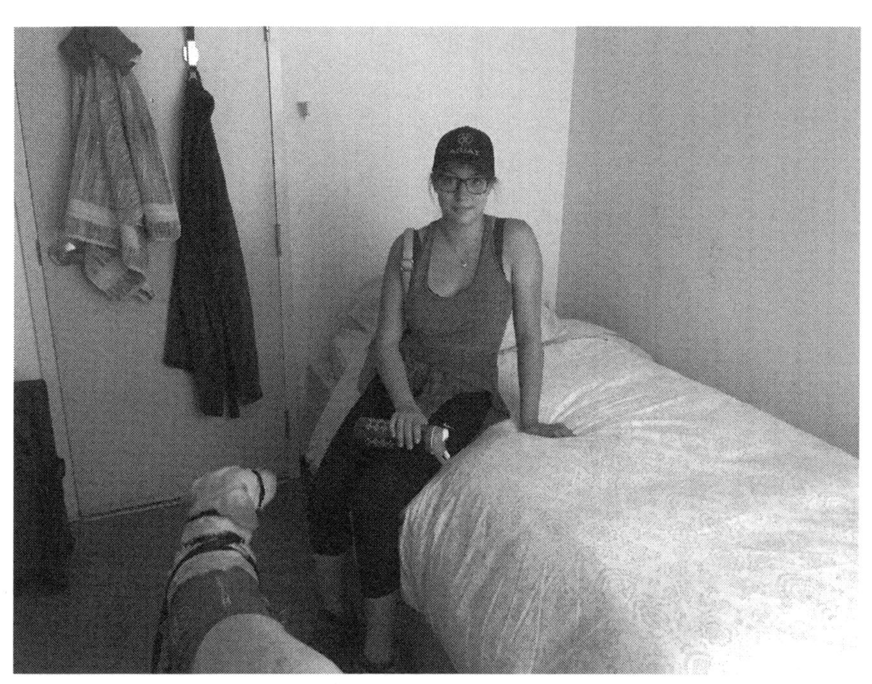

Zandra in her room at the University of Victoria

CHAPTER 14

When Things Got Worse

THE FALL OF 2018 STARTED off on a high. My trip to Tanzania was nothing short of spectacular. Fulfilling a lifelong dream for me was an extraordinary feat. It was an experience I had dreamt of before I stopped allowing myself to dream. This trip was something I had seen myself doing in one of my earliest visions of my future self, before I ever saw myself married or having children. I needed to do this for myself, yet the reasons were still unknown.

Elephants have always been special to me. My love of elephants began early on. I remember watching a nature show on TV and seeing how female elephants surround each other to form a protection within their community. These females were usually gentle giants, yet when they needed to be they could fiercely protect themselves and each other. When a baby was orphaned the other mothers would take over, providing safety and protection. Elephants are also known for their memory. Not only can they recognize all the members of their own clan, but any others, including humans, who have left a great impression on them.

I always felt connected to elephants in an unexplainable way, as if I had been amongst them in a different time. In my own young life, I wished for an elephant-like tribe: a fierce clan I could rely on to protect me, a clan who would rally around me when I was hurt or scared. My admiration for these magnificent animals was reaffirmed once I saw them in person. I stood in awe as I watched, with my own eyes, the relationships and behaviours that I had only ever seen on TV. As I stood amongst the other wild women whose dreams had also taken them to this place, I realized that we formed our own tribes. I may not belong to their clans, but the beautiful souls I met left a lifelong impression with me. As I camped and travelled through Tanzania, I had an inner knowledge that my experience would feed my soul for the rest of my life. Sometimes when I can't sleep, I recall the herd of zebras that ran into the Maasai village that I was camping in, causing a lot of ruckus and excitement, or the sound of the elephants, quietly walking along the back of my tent as I heard the sound of a trunk rubbing across the canvas. In these moments I felt as wild as the animals, and a part of their kingdom.

Shortly after I returned home, before I had even fully recovered from my jetlag, the ground came out from under me. When I left for Africa, Gord's law practice was doing very well. So well, in fact, that we had decided we would both upgrade our vehicles. Life was feeling like it was at a high point. My instinct was telling me that something was coming, but I had no idea what. I quelled my gut by telling myself that we deserved good things, and after such a rough year we should be open to them, yet the feeling still nagged.

Gord called me with news: he'd had a contract that was suddenly terminated, one that provided for over half of his income at the time. We felt destroyed. There was no way for us to foresee this problem or stop it from happening. We needed to come together as a family and make some big changes. In a perverse way I felt relieved. I had known something was coming for several months and now it had arrived. The monster in the closet is much more frightening when you dread it than when you open the door and see it. I had an understanding that whenever things happened, no matter how uncomfortable or scary they were, I was never alone. I always put my faith in God and knew that He uses difficult times to grow me. In this case, it was my family. We needed to circle around one another. Like the elephants in Africa, we needed to provide a safe place for our children. We had no idea how long it would take to recoup our losses but knew that the new cars needed to go. Even though we took a steep financial loss, we traded them in for vehicles that we owned without payments. We were not sure if our next step would be a move. I loved my house, yet in that moment I could easily see myself being equally happy in another downsized home. Nothing mattered to me more than the wellbeing of my family, and when things get tough they get surprisingly simple.

My mind wandered to the reasons for what was occurring. There are no accidents, this was meant to happen, yet in the turmoil I was blind to the lesson. I never felt lost—somehow I knew this was a rebirth for me—but the stress took its toll as well. One lesson that stood out clearly for us both was to always be prepared. We failed, like many people, to have enough money set aside for such a crisis. Although we were well insured and had been carefully planning for our future retirements, we lacked an emergency fund to support ourselves over several months. We scrambled to cut our expenses.

Amongst the mounding stress, there were several gifts. Gord and I learned that when put to the test, we valued the same things. Both of us are hard workers and would do anything to support our family. During the crisis, we learned to communicate in an even deeper way. We also knew that this lesson was something for the entire family. The children needed to know that this was life. Bad things happen and the sun will always come up again. In such times, we need to pull even closer to family, friends and community rather than isolate and allow our fears to consume us. This was raw and real, and we were appreciative that we could demonstrate that, no matter what happened, we would pull through.

Although Zandra lived away from us, she was very much a part of our group. We let her know of the uncertainty and included her in the team building. We didn't want her to stress, even when for several months we felt certain we might lose our home. Through all of this she was supportive and positive. I looked forward to her texts showing dense green forests and ocean views. It appeared that she and Cinnamon were exploring daily and getting to know their new city. Zandra hadn't taken her car to the Island. It was too expensive to park at the university, so she ended up walking a lot. For the times she needed to go farther, she went outside of her comfort zone and learned the bus routes, something she couldn't wait to share with me in one of our discussions.

Living in university residence was a benefit in many ways. Zandra was a close walk to the buildings she needed and could easily return Cinnamon to her room for the chemistry labs that she couldn't attend. On the flip side, the dormitory building grew to life on the weekends, filled with teenagers drinking and partying. Zandra had never been a part of that crowd, not even in high school. She felt isolated in her room, listening to all the groups of kids having fun, feeling lonelier than ever. At least in her condo she could bake and move about, and she had her own bathroom. Another stress for her was the food service. The cafeterias catered to the freshmen crowd, serving feasts of burgers, fries and pasta. These were meals that caused large spikes in blood sugars and were composed of foods that she's intolerant to and had avoided most of her life. It became increasingly difficult for her to make wise dietary choices.

When Christmas came, we were excited to have her come home. Some of my conversations with her were becoming increasingly reminiscent of the types of calls we shared while she was living in Edmonton, when I was concerned for her mental and physical wellbeing. She was lonely and her blood sugars were often high. She had told me that she was reverting to the old "Netflix and eating," as well as overcorrecting for her lows in the night. She was beginning to spiral downwards, and the holidays couldn't have come at a better time. I couldn't wait to have her amongst her family and friends. She needed to reset and the break was timely.

While she was home, her blood sugars were as terrible as I feared, despite how she was eating. I hadn't seen such high blood sugars since her diagnosis. "When did they start getting so high?" I asked when she appeared okay with it. I was angry that she seemed so cavalier about her levels. I should have known that she was not at all comfortable with the blood sugars as she began to sob. "I don't feel well. I'm not doing well in school, although I'm passing, and my body is letting me down." I didn't know what to do for her. I could see for myself how off the rails she looked. She was lonely, had dangerously high blood sugars and was struggling emotionally. I didn't want to send her back.

The Christmas break flew by quickly. Although I worked through a lot of it, I managed to spend some quality time with Zandra. We walked dogs along the golf course, watched *Anne of Green Gables* and made a lot of healthy vegan meals that she enjoyed. Zandra had an appointment with the adult diabetes clinic in Edmonton a few days before she left. I wasn't able to go with her as I had a heavy work schedule, so she went alone. When she returned, she was in tears. She was told that the blood test she had taken prior to her appointment showed her highest ever A1C, and her thyroid was functioning even lower. She had shown the nurse her shin again, yet they couldn't determine the cause, and, in Zandra's opinion, seemed unwilling to do further investigations. She felt dismissed and disheartened.

Zandra had to leave that Sunday afternoon to get back for class the following morning. Our plan was to go to church as a family and I would drive her to the airport afterwards. The night before, I was really struggling to let her go. She wasn't okay and neither was I. How could things have become so bleak when just months ago I was in Africa, feeling on top of the world? I realized that there was something I could do. I asked Zandra if she wanted to leave church early so we could go to the office and do a hypnotherapy session before she left. She was all in. In the morning I woke up early to get everything I needed ready. I knew exactly what suggestions she needed, and most importantly I believed wholeheartedly that she had what it took to heal herself of her stress. The session was beautiful and peaceful. She felt amazing afterwards, and a few days later the suggestions I made were confirmed to have made a difference. For the first time in many weeks she was starting to test in the normal ranges. Unfortunately, it didn't hold.

I had begun to keep my phone on throughout the night again, like I had the previous year, so Zandra could call or text if she needed. The frequency of her calls was increasing and often continued throughout the night. Things had never been so difficult. Zandra's blood sugars refused to go down despite the insulin she used. Several times she tested positive for ketones and would have to manually inject insulin to be sure there wasn't a fault with her pump. I was racking my brain to come up with reasons for her high blood sugars. I considered whether it was a faulty pump, her emotional state, her insulin being overheated or expired, or anything else that could explain her dangerously high numbers. Everywhere I went, the grocery store or one of the children's activities, diabetes was on my mind. It was interfering with my sleep, work and relationships with my other children. At least the financial stresses were lifting in our home life. Gord was working extremely hard and had managed to not only bounce back, but put money away so if we ever were in another crisis we would have some resources.

The university broke in February for reading week, a time for students to rest and recuperate from the stresses of the academic pressures. These breaks are designed by the institutions to acknowledge that when a student is under academic pressure, combined with other stress factors, they are at a risk of suicide. Things had become so difficult for Zandra that I felt I needed to see her. I booked a flight and headed out at the beginning of her break. Both Zandra and Cinnamon were excited to see me, and I was met with lots of tight hugs and canine kisses. We decided to spend the first night together in her dorm room so I could get the full experience of her life in residence.

Zandra had graciously given me her single bed, while she and Cinnamon took to the floor. It was tight, but a lot of fun. Victoria had experienced a historic snowfall just a week prior to my arrival. Snow on the Island is heavy and slippery and very dangerous. The roads had become impossible to drive, and many businesses and schools were closed. The evidence of snowfall was still on the ground when I arrived, although much of it had melted already. Underneath the snow were the signs of spring. The smell of green grass and damp ground was refreshing compared to the still-freezing winter temperatures back home. We walked on one of her favourite trails by the school and came back to the cafeteria for supper. I followed Zandra and Cinnamon along as they grabbed a tray and walked along to the menu posted on the wall. Zandra was excited because they were serving falafel burgers, something we both liked. I was touched by the way she greeted the cashier and servers. They all knew her by name. Zandra sticks out from a crowd most of the time because a vested dog accompanies her, but this was different. She really knew these people and they knew her.

We walked along the length of the serving aisle as we had our plates filled with burgers and salad. We walked to the cups and filled ours with water from the dispenser. Zandra ushered me toward her usual table where she liked to sit by herself, a place that is quiet yet allows Cinnamon some room so as not to be stepped on by the other students.

Once we sat down, I asked her about the workers that she seemed to know. She explained that, "The lady who served our burgers likes to rock climb and has climbed a lot of peaks in her time." She often chatted with Zandra about where to hike and climb in the area. The lady at the till was more of a motherly sort. "She lives farther away and has a daughter who is a student. She gives great advice and we even exchanged valentine gifts!" My heart melted. This was my kid. She sees people. I watched as dozens of other students, the ones who remained during the break, walk through and not give so much as a thank you. I was glad my daughter was different. These faces were her friends. They were the faces of the tribe that she had made for herself.

While we were eating, we got talking about the other meals that were provided in the cafeteria. I asked her about the buns we were eating—I had assumed they were gluten-free. She indicated they were full-wheat buns. "Gluten-free is hard to come by and you get what you get at the end of the day," she said. I was alarmed. Zandra had never digested wheat properly. I felt I had stumbled on part of the problem. I knew that, although it would be hard, she had to stop eating wheat. The meal was quite good, considering that it was from a cafeteria, and after supper we walked back to her room to cozy up and have girls' night in.

The following morning was dewy and fresh. I was thrilled to see rain after so many months, so we decided to head out for a walk. The ocean was a short trip from campus, so we headed down the main road, which passes the little shop she worked at on the way. Zandra had taken a job at Pepper's Grocery, a neighbourhood grocery store, where she was hired in the meat department. Her job was to cut and package meat. She had hoped to be hired as a cashier, but the only opening they had was in the meat department. With some free time on her hands and no real friends, she felt she could get a job to cover some of her expenses. Having a vegan work in the meat department was a joke in our own family, although she tried not to let on at the store for fear of being teased.

The beach was refreshing and filled with dogs and their owners. This was clearly one of Zandra's favourite places to be. She recognized most of the dogs and was friendly with their owners. This was another place she belonged in. We watched Cinnamon play in the water for a while, marvelling at how many beaches she has had the privilege to dip her tail into in her lifetime. The day felt normal and needed, yet the undertones of despair were as thick as the fog in the air. This visit was a temporary patch and wouldn't last long.

After our walk, we went to check in to our accommodations. It was an original homestead property with a historic house along the Patricia Bay Highway. The host was exceptional and very personable. She greeted Cinnamon as a special guest, with a dog bed and dishes set out in advance. We were excited to have a bed that we could stretch out in and enjoy a bathroom to ourselves. We would only be there a few nights, and already time seemed to be closing in. We vowed to make the most of it, so we planned out the other places we hoped to go. The manager at Pepper's coached a ladies' soccer league and had lost his goalie partway through the season. When he found out that Zandra had experience, he recruited her as a fill-in. There wasn't much of the season left, but that evening there was a game on the west side of town. I hadn't seen a soccer game in several years and was thrilled to watch her play after so long away from the game.

The drizzly rain had turned into a gentle snow by the start of the game that evening. The field was at a school that had artificial turf but no spectator benches. I had planned for the cool weather and bundled up with my winter coat, mitts and toque. I had also brought a blanket for Cinnamon that I intended for her to lie on, but when I noticed her shivering I draped it across her like a cape instead. The game was fun to watch, but by the end Zandra's team had lost and we were all too cold to care. I enjoyed being able to watch Zandra as she ran across the net and blocked most of the balls that came her way.

During the night I watched Zandra get up several times to test. Each time she did, she was extremely high and needed to correct with large amounts of insulin. I couldn't imagine the stress she was under, not to mention how ill she must have felt. I watched everything she ate, yet the blood sugars wouldn't go down. I wanted to break down and cry. I had a strong desire to shut down and give in to my frustration, but I couldn't. She needed me to be strong. She needed me to encourage her to press on and believe things would change.

The next day we had decided to head downtown. I had missed being with her for her birthday the month prior and we had decided to find a gift in the Lush store on Government Street. Zandra had picked out her favourite rose body spray as her gift. It was a beautiful scent, sweet and strong like the girl it was intended for. We opted out of purchasing a bag and decided my purse was large enough for it until we got back to the room. After our shopping was finished, we went out for supper before heading back. Once we returned to our place, I went to pull out the body spray and discovered that the bottle sprayer had worked itself loose and spilled half the contents into my purse, which now smelled strongly of rose. I felt terrible that I had ruined her gift. To make up for the mishap, we decided to see an IMAX show. The Alex Honnold film *Free Solo* was playing and interested us both. As I went to the counter to pay for our tickets, the clerk acknowledged, "Rose body spray from Lush?" I hadn't realized until then how much I reeked of rose!

The film had us on the edge of our seats as we watched Alex scale heights that nobody had before. We realized that the people in front of us moved seats part way through the show—likely because of the strong odour emanating from my purse. We laughed as we realized that even we were getting headaches.

The following day was the last of my visit. I had to leave after breakfast and return Zandra and Cinnamon to the university before heading to the airport. I tried to keep upbeat, and although Zandra tried as well, she cried throughout the morning. We packed up our things and headed back to the dorms. I only had ten minutes to say goodbye while we sorted out her things from mine. I asked Zandra to switch purses with me so as not to bother anyone on the plane. She hardly ever used a purse, so she hung mine up on the back of the door to use as an air freshener. Saying goodbye was even harder this time. I knew she wasn't well, and I still had to leave her. She didn't have anything fun to look forward to, as midterm exams were only days away. Before I departed we hugged, and as I pulled away I watched Zandra standing and crying with Cinnamon from my rear-view mirror.

At the airport I pulled out my wallet. I could smell the rose scent that had soaked the leather; it had me in tears. I couldn't stop. I spent the flight home dabbing my eyes as my body fought leaving Zandra behind.

Zandra passed her midterms, but by no means excelled. She was spending her nights awake trying to control her blood sugars and her days trying to cope. She had been in contact with the diabetes clinic in Edmonton for months, trying to get help from a distance. There wasn't a lot they could do unless she needed acute care. It seemed to them that she was becoming intolerant to insulin. If that were the case, serious intervention would be needed. We considered pulling her out of school—it was becoming a matter of life and death. Her body would not be able to sustain the high blood sugars for much longer. Often times her sugars were so high they were unreadable to her tester. She was beginning to look as sick as she felt.

Instead of improving, things only got worse. After a long night of having Zandra on the phone stressed that her blood sugars wouldn't budge, I had to head off to Calgary for a work conference. At this time I was working for an organization that recognizes the increasing youth suicide rate, and offered a community-based program to identify those at need and support them. After spending endless weeks supporting Zandra and the other kids and working with youth suicide, I was burnt out. I needed the trip away, but instead of working I wanted to throw the blankets over my head and not come up for days. The clouds grew heavy as I drove to Calgary. I could see that I would pass through sleet, strong winds and slippery roads. The storm clouds reflected the heaviness of my thoughts as I began praying out loud for help. I begged for a sign that there was hope and relief for Zandra. I needed to find my centre so I could keep going.

When I checked in to my hotel room it was nearly four in the afternoon. I decided I was too exhausted to go anywhere to eat, so I resigned myself to the complimentary black tea and the bag of baby carrots I had brought from home. I turned on the TV and recognized the old show *Touched by an Angel*. The episode was almost over as the angel, Monica, played by Roma Downing, was beginning to speak. What I caught was ". . . God didn't give you diabetes, but he did give you everything you need to live with it. He gave you the right doctors and the right medicine, and the right family. He gave you something else, too. Every time you have to take a shot, or test your blood, or even think about this disease, you'll remember how fragile life is, and you'll wake up every morning thanking your creator for still being alive, something not everyone does."

I couldn't believe it. I was looking around my hotel room in shock, as if an angel would appear to me in real life. I was the only one in the room that I could see, yet I didn't feel alone. Then the angel spoke to the mother in the show, saying, "You can't carry this burden for Amy [the daughter with diabetes], and she doesn't need you to." Tears started flowing without control. I didn't know what to make of it. The words were meant for me and were exactly what I needed to hear.

I hadn't realized how much of a burden I was shouldering until that moment. Somehow, along the way I chose to try to control a disease that wasn't mine. My motives were pure, yet not effective for any of us. Any parent would want to take the disease for their child. I wanted to make life normal for Zandra so she could know the carefree life that every child deserves. As her mother, it was my job to care for her, yet somehow in the caring I had taken full control.

As I sat on the bed with my bag of carrots spilling out of the bag, I realized that God gave her diabetes, not me. My mind raced as I tried to decipher the message like Morse code. I couldn't begin to understand how to let go—how to pull back yet still support her. Then it started to become clear. At some point, a counsellor needs to empower their client to answer their own questions from within, to always empower the individual in their own life but be there for support when they needed. As a parent, I knew that the same rules applied. Somehow, in my fear I had taken over. God knows and loves Zandra, too. He knew she could handle this disease and He knew that I could support her. I needed to let go and let God lead.

I grabbed my phone and texted Zandra. I knew that she might get something from this message as well, albeit in her own perspective. I looked up and sent her the YouTube link for season 6, episode 20, and asked her to watch it when she had a chance. She returned my text an hour later and replied with a heartfelt message that had it not been for the cheesy aspects of the old show, she would have been crying. She appreciated the message and was heartened to see diabetes portrayed on a show.

I had a hard time sleeping that evening. My mind was turning over and over. But, overall, I felt a deep sense of love. My prayers had been heard and I knew that, whatever the outcome, I walked with God, in purpose.

CHAPTER 15

Finding Purpose in Letting Go

When the new semester started in January, Zandra shared a math class with an outgoing blond girl named Abby. Throughout the year I had heard her speak of a couple of school acquaintances, but nobody she would call a friend. More and more I was hearing of Abby during our calls, realizing that she was becoming her first true friend in a long time. It had been so long since I had heard her talk about going out with a friend it sounded like music to my ears. Zandra had a lighter, easier sense about her. I was elated that her wish for a friend came true. More and more when I would call or text, she would be busy and would need to return my call. Abby was a breath of fresh air. Zandra described her as tall, naturally slim, and beautiful from the inside out. She had a sense of herself and an openness to connect with others easily, something Zandra admired. Abby lived alone in a small basement suite not far from campus. Zandra discovered that they both had little red cars, each named after flowers: Zandra's was Rosie and Abby's was Poppy.

When Zandra wasn't with Abby, she found herself mired in the same old patterns of thinking and behaving. She feared loneliness, which propelled her to "Netflix and eat." When this happened, she would spiral down a well-worn path of shame, fear and regret. To Zandra, Abby appeared to have no troubles of her own, something I quickly debunked. I encouraged her to talk to Abby about her problems, so she felt she had someone around her who understood and increased her support at the same time. Although it took a while, she finally confessed her troubles to Abby. Abby, like a true friend, listened to Zandra and offered support for when she needed it. This cemented the friendship. I felt a peace knowing that Zandra had other supports in place and that she was learning to be open about her own struggles.

Ever since my experience in the hotel room, I took the message to heart. I guided as many conversations as I could for Zandra to listen to her own intuition, to see what she needed from her own soul before she consulted with anyone else. I could see her repeating my own patterns of holding shame and rarely opening up about the very intimate struggles that I'd faced. I explained to her that we are more connected to others by our grief than we are in any other way. I began to see her slowly opening, like a rosebud in the sun.

After school was over for the year, Zandra decided to come home for the summer. She got a job with the county, cutting grass and working outside, which paid a generous wage to students. By the end of the year she was happy to never sleep in a dorm room again. She had planned to look for a place for the upcoming school year with Abby and drive up with her car, so she had it at her disposal. The summer was looking bright with hope and promise.

Zandra had taken my advice and stopped eating wheat again, even though it left her with very few options for the remaining months while living in residence. In addition to wheat, she eliminated most processed foods, including processed grains, which removed the option of even gluten-free bread. Although she was still experiencing spikes in her blood sugar levels that were unexplained, the frequency had drastically reduced from just a month prior and it seemed that she was no longer in a dangerous situation. While at home, I made sure to support her health with a lot of vegan meals. Zandra liked to start off her days with a run before work and before the heat of the day set in. Cinnamon was slowing down, and running a few miles was no longer something she could easily do with arthritis starting to settle in, so she would take our family dog, Axel, along with her. Axel is a Border Collie–Great Pyrenees cross. He's got long legs and a trim body, perfect for a running companion; however, his thick black and white spotted coat makes overheating a problem. Luckily, the mornings were usually cool, and they enjoyed sharing this start to each day with each other.

As the running progressed, so did the pain in Zandra's shin. The existing sores were now becoming an even deeper shade of red and starting to bleed as well. The pain was getting unbearable at times, most often during and after a run. Whenever I suggested she slow down or take a few days' respite, she was determined not to let anything stop her. I could see the old drill sergeant coming out in her, and the frustration and anger at her body surfacing, repeating the feelings that had been lying dormant for the past months.

I was very concerned about the bruises, and I suspected that Zandra's recent behaviour was an indication that she was concerned as well. Nobody seemed to know what to do. When Zandra last saw her general physician, he prescribed an antibiotic cream. He always felt that it was diabetes-related, yet the doctors and nurses at the clinic felt it wasn't related at all. Frustrated with the system, Zandra had decided to go back to our family paediatrician, Dr. Dhunnoo. He suggested that she had some sort of ulcer but didn't specialize in diabetes to know how to best treat it. After expressing his own frustration that we still didn't have answers, he referred her to a bone specialist. The appointment wouldn't be until later in the summer, but hopefully we would have some answers before she left for school in the fall. In the meanwhile he could offer her little, other than to suggest she listen to her body about what she could and could not do.

Zandra continued to run through her pain. She suffered through the agony and continued to regularly punish her body. Each step would exacerbate her symptoms. She complained, yet refused to alter her routine. What should have been a run to support her health was instead punishing it. As much as I enjoyed having all the children at home, I was struggling to watch the display of anger and fury. I was slipping into my own despair, not sure how or when this would end.

Finally, with summer coming to a close, the specialist appointment came. She went with her cousin Gillian, as they were already together in Edmonton on the day of the appointment. Gillian was planning to drive to the Island with her early the next morning. She was joining Zandra for the adventure of a cross-provincial trip and the company, so she had someone to be with.

The doctor was running a few minutes late, but promptly gave his diagnosis. He diagnosed her with necrobiosis lipoidica, a condition that is thought to be linked to blood-vessel inflammation related to autoimmune factors, mostly affecting those with type 1 diabetes. The condition is rare and has no proven cure. The doctor immediately ordered Zandra to discontinue any aerobic exercise, indicating to her that it may be indefinitely. He offered no supports, medicines or options beyond that and sent her on her way until the results of her bone scan came back which would determine the amount of damage to her shin.

When Zandra came home from the appointment with Gillian, she wouldn't talk. I asked her how it went and she flew upstairs, with silent torment, to her room, leaving Gillian to answer my questions. Gillian explained that the doctor had very little bedside manner. He was rude and unsympathetic to a young person hearing the diagnosis. His lack of empathy and support was deeply upsetting to Zandra and she clearly didn't know how to cope with it.

After talking to Gillian, I went into Zandra's room to offer encouragement and support, but she shut me down. She wasn't ready for the bright side that I would try to spin. She sent me out of her room. For quite some time she had used running as a control for her blood sugars. She was unwilling to relent and now she was forced to. I did my best not to carry this burden, not to take it over and try to make it all better. She had her own struggles and I had mine. I knew in my own life that anger was a blessing. It motivated me to ask questions, to seek answers and push through the heaviness of my own heart. I knew that if I allowed her time, she just may receive the same blessing.

The next day we said goodbye. I was planning on meeting up with them soon, however. After Zandra and I went to Iceland, Gord and I decided to start a tradition: when the kids become teenagers, they get to pick a destination for a trip with me. Zandra's was Iceland, Olivia had chosen Houston, Texas, and now it was Joseph's turn. He chose Seattle, Washington because he wanted to bring Zandra and Devin along, and knew it was close to Victoria. We had a wonderful time together despite the diagnosis just days before. But I knew the pain would surface again.

Zandra began her classes and her life was off to a much better start. Although it was a challenge to find a suite that would allow Cinnamon, Abby had searched tirelessly and found one. Early in the first semester, Zandra realized that she didn't feel her program was for her. She explained that the biology classes weren't what she thought they would be—she wanted to know more about human systems. She wanted to change her major to encompass a wider range of career opportunities. She had expressed that after her degree, she wanted to consider going into medicine. This was another step in the direction she felt called to. I liked to joke that while her experience cutting meat at Pepper's didn't help her appetite, it might have prepared her for medical school!

After a couple of weeks, she met with an academic advisor and had her schedule switched. It was clear that she was tapping into her intuition more and more, seeking what her heart was calling her to do. Still, there were many ups and downs with her diabetes. With every cold and flu, her blood sugars swung into uncontrollably high levels that created stress on her mind and body. Zandra has always deeply cared about the long-term implications of poorly controlled blood sugars. The expectation that blood sugars are something that can be *controlled* can often be frustrating to those with diabetes and their helpers. Exam stress, boyfriend trouble, illness and even the time of day can all result in unpredictable levels. Often the only control is in doing the best you can and then relinquishing it for a spell.

CHAPTER 16

Walk of Faith

As I write this book, Zandra is going into her fourth year of studying science at university. Together we have walked a journey that has led us on rugged terrain more often than smooth pavement. Many of the greatest memories of my life have been shared while walking alongside her as we both learned about ourselves through her struggles with diabetes. Each twist and turn in the road has provided me with greater perspective than I would have known otherwise. It seems strange to say that I'm grateful for diabetes, yet in a way I am. I wouldn't want to go back to the person I was before Zandra's diagnosis. I have a deeper meaning in my life and a love of myself that I never knew possible.

I am deeply proud of how Zandra has worked so hard to lead a healthy and full life despite her struggles. This past fall, Zandra experienced lower back pain and assumed it was an injury from working out at the gym. The pain seemed to be manageable for a while, until early November. After riding horses with Abby, she realized that her pain was something worse than sore muscles. Abby went with Zandra to a medical clinic where she was diagnosed immediately with a kidney infection.

The infection cleared up with antibiotics; however, her routine bloodwork throughout the following months revealed that her kidney function was impaired. While Zandra was home for the Christmas break, she had a routine exam with her doctor. He sent her home with another blood requisition, which showed that things were getting worse. Her doctor emailed her yet another requisition for her to do on Christmas Eve, warning that if the results didn't get any better, she would be admitted to the hospital and possibly put on dialysis.

The fear for Zandra and our entire family made for a holiday that cared little for the typical holiday fare and focused instead on the real aspects of gathering. Everyone, including our extended family, friends, and the church, openly shared prayers and sent love her way. When she went for her final test on Christmas Eve, there was no trace of kidney problems. It was a Christmas miracle. When I reflect back on that experience, I realize that we were all in God's hands, no matter what the outcome would have been. I felt myself surrender to a greater source and actively worked at releasing my own fear.

Whatever Zandra's next steps are, I know that she desires to be a support for those who struggle with diabetes. She has progressed from paralyzing fear of people knowing of her diabetes to actively seeking out those who may benefit from her experience and support. I hold a prayer in my heart that a cure for diabetes can be found before any other parent or child experiences the need to inject insulin in order to live, yet I know that the timing of that is completely out of my control.

While I wait for my prayer to be answered, I know that diabetes is on the rise. Over 300,000 Canadians are living with type 1 diabetes, which affects every individual and their families in different ways. Sadly, like Ty, there are many who pass of complications each year. The grief felt by those family members who loved and supported a child with diabetes only to lose them is the ultimate tragedy. For each parent, nothing could be more devastating as they mourn the loss of their loved one. Each loss robs a parent of the relationship that they held visions of since the beginning of their child's life. For anyone who has experienced a loss of any kind, I am deeply sorry for it and carry your burden with you. Every life has immense meaning, whether they are here or departed.

The way to move forward is only found in the absence of fear. Every life is a beautiful story that has the potential to enrich those who had the privilege to be touched by them in some way. Each person touched by the life light of another becomes an even brighter vessel who can carry the memories of those they hold dear. As Albert Einstein revealed,

"Energy cannot be created or destroyed, it can only be changed from one form into another." The spirit and energy of those we lose will always be near. I believe that the support from those who struggled in this life supports the others and their families from the other side. This strongly held belief gives me great encouragement when I have feared losing my own child to this disease.

Each struggle, whether it belongs to me or to someone close to me, has proven to be a valuable life lesson for me. In the moment, that struggle feels like a curse, as if I've been punished and tested. This feeling has led me down many dark roads, which have only further led me astray. In that state, the notion that despair can lead me to deepen my understanding and awareness of love feels simply absurd. It has taken multiple events followed often by much distress to teach me that if I believe there is a purpose in my life, my old ways would have never led me to my higher purpose.

Every time I faced any adversity I labelled myself as unworthy, fostering a belief that I wasn't enough. Every success that I achieved was motivated by proving my feelings of inadequacy wrong. My fight for approval only anchored these beliefs after living this way for many years. These beliefs contorted my view of the world to a place I no longer wanted to exist in. Joy became unfamiliar to me, and the lack of it became normal.

I am learning that I hold the control for how I choose to see things in my life. I spent far too much time feeling as though I was unworthy, that I wasn't good enough, and the worst: that something would invariably go wrong. My sensitivity to feeling everything became my fear of feeling anything. What I showed on the outside was an act. I put on my happy face when I held my baby for the camera. The love was real, but the fear that was equally present was hidden, except to me. I always felt like a fraud and was scared to be found out. I knew that I was hiding a part of myself in the fear of being exposed. I was afraid that I would be judged and my unworthiness would become even heavier. What I didn't know at the time was that I was robbing myself of the support that was all around me, support that was ready to help if only I acted out of love instead of fear.

When Zandra was born I was already primed to see through my distorted looking glass. I lacked the self-love to live from my true self, love that allows feelings to be fully present in the moment and forgives mistakes along the way. I allowed every unfair comment to keep me feeling victim to my own situation and prevent me from feeling peace and joy. I didn't do this on purpose; it bypassed every check and balance within my consciousness and activated my core beliefs. I felt prisoner to my old stories and, although I didn't see myself as a victim, I felt enslaved by every negative experience, all at the same time.

When Zandra was diagnosed with diabetes, my deeply rooted fear that something bad was going to happen, something out of my control, was triggered. My long-held belief came to fruition and I set into action mode to triage the situation. I was a pro at sorting through the rubble of a bad situation and pulling out pieces of hope. I spent that first night after Zandra's diagnosis looking for ways in which to find meaning for her and the hand she was dealt. My sense of purpose was heightened in moments like this and I became very adept at handling crises. Because of my early life, I learned to actively seek out the positives and hand out hope in bad situations to appease others' discomfort. I did this selfishly, as when others felt better, so did I. Their discomfort was my discomfort. I knew I was good at that, yet that high from helping would soon fizzle out and I'd be back to where I started. I was wrong to believe that my role was to solve others' problems or search for the meaning in their lives, instead of guiding them to see it for themselves.

If anyone would have asked me years ago what my purpose in this life was, I would respond that I was meant to give comfort to those when their confidence was down. My intentions were pure and my motives free from ego. I had a genuine desire to help, and because I was very empathic I could feel the difference I made. When it came to Zandra's diagnosis, my genuine desire to help her see that she was bigger than any disease came from a place of love and a belief that her precious life held immense value, yet I lacked the understanding that the disease was also for me. On an intellectual level, I understood that in order to give you must first possess that which you wish to give away, yet I didn't see myself as lacking. It wasn't until I began to provide advice, advice that

I knew I needed to follow for myself, that I understood this at a much deeper level.

In my role as a parent, I have realized that I have been personally challenged, match for match. In order to coach the next skill, I had to make sure I understood the test inside out. My greatest strength has been the insight to understand my challenge and face each fear head on. The lessons I have learned have been unequivocally more than I could have ever been taught in any other way than by immersion. I know that the path has been equally meaningful for Zandra, yet I can say with utmost certainty that her struggles have enriched my life. If I had to choose the enlightenment from this journey over my pain, I would choose enlightenment every time, although that observation is much easier in hindsight.

In this life we have no guarantees. My life would have been made much simpler had I known the happy ever after of my own perspective would actually be my final outcome. If that were the case, I would race through the events of my life, never taking in the deeper meaning that my struggles have shown me. Instead, all we have is faith. I have no guarantees that diabetes won't devastate my life. I have no guarantees that I won't have to watch Zandra, or either one of my children, struggle, or, even worse, lose them. The very thought evokes fear in my being. When these thoughts become intrusive, or a reality, I know I am called to hold faith that the hand of God is in everything and working through me, and every one of us, for the greater good. As a result of my experiences, I now allow God to guide me as I become open to all possibilities and move further away from my own desired outcomes. If we believe we are full of value and that everything we do has meaning, then we open ourselves to greater possibilities that are perhaps more spectacular than anything our minds could ever conceive of.

I am aware that in the last several years my mind has taken a great shift away from the way it used to be. As I practice being open to possibility, even in the most difficult times, possibilities quickly becoming much clearer. I'm able to reduce the stress in my life and realize that every setback I experience is a challenge intended for my greater good. This is not to say I don't experience sadness or get fearful at times; rather, it allows me to experience those emotions and move beyond them, recognizing that I have the choice to be in fear or move forward out of love. When I fully allow the creativity of God, I am able to glimpse the worst of my fears and know that I am and will always be able to face my doubts and find a deeper meaning in them.

In my experience I have found that at times the effort to transform my entire way of thinking into openness has been deeply exhausting. In my darkest days I have felt depleted of the energy required to be openly aware of my experiences. I've always felt a sense of urgency in my life that has at times helped me to move forward quickly, but I can lose hope if I don't. Perhaps one of the greatest lessons, one I'm still discovering, is that there is no set timeline to realizing how to move forward. Knowing this allows us the most humility. It is where I learned to open myself to receiving rather than always giving. When I've taken my time and fully explored my emotions, I've learned to allow myself to be the one supported by others. Most often this includes my husband and children. This in turn has allowed them to realize that they have the insight, empathy and nurturing necessary to help others as well.

Several synchronicities have transpired over the last year to inspire me to write about my experiences with having a diabetic child. The first was something that levelled the landscape of my life. It cleared the way for the building of not only this book, but also a much greater understanding of myself. I was fired. I had been working in a job that I loved, supporting youth at risk for suicide. It was a job that I was good at and knew it. Unfortunately, I spoke out against the mistreatment of a therapy dog in our care named Moose and was terminated for the effort.

During this time, Zandra was struggling as well. When she would call, I felt as though I could offer her little. I could no longer hold myself as an example of how to serve others—I felt as though I had failed. I struggled to see how I could be a role model for Zandra when I felt as though I was left without purpose. I needed to challenge myself to take hold of everything I had learned and be the example of how to move forward. From the moment I spoke out about Moose's care and lost my job, I felt that I was on autopilot. I had a sense deep within me that I had to follow my values. My integrity was more valuable than my pride. Although speaking up for a voiceless animal triggered the events that led to my dismissal, I knew I had to do it, and I don't regret any of it.

In the months that passed, I found that standing within my integrity was a lonely place. I had friends and family who supported me, yet inside I felt entirely alone. I had no idea of my next steps, yet I felt I had a calling, something bigger than I could recognize. Gord was of great support during this time and encouraged me take the time to discover new interests and pursue other goals. He had seen how drained I had become managing the fears of Zandra's blood sugars and he saw the break as a blessing for me. During this time, I began to receive even more support from Zandra, who in turn was using her own lessons from her life to demonstrate to me how to move forward with my own. She spoke of how often she felt like she was alone with something she didn't know how to manage, yet challenged herself to bring out her greatest callings. She encouraged me by saying that my work to help others had only begun, and inspired me with stories of how I had helped her so often when she was fearful of her future.

About a month after I was let go from my job, I woke up in the middle of the night with the calling to write a book. This calling was clear and planted in my mind like the answer to a long-awaited mystery. It was as if I was looking at something for the first time yet knowing it had been there all along. I lay awake for some time pondering the idea, yet dismissed it with the light of the following day. The idea kept coming back to me with every moment of quiet. It seeped into my dreams and into my thoughts. I kept challenging the idea, dismissing it with the knowledge that I was not a writer and completely out of my depth. But God was persistent.

I felt called to read the Bible. I had never really read the Bible, opting instead to listen to readings and sermons at church. The same desire that called me to speak up for Moose inspired me to read the Bible. I soon came across the story of Moses being asked by God to talk to the slaves. Moses resisted the request, acknowledging that he wasn't as capable as his brother Aaron at speaking to large crowds. He asked God to call upon his brother to fulfill the request. God spoke to Moses and told him that it was he whom the people needed to hear from. He was instructed that he could use his brother to help him convey his message. They were a team, and each as valuable as the other.

This message resonated within me. My fear of not being a professional writer and feeling inadequate was something that God could overlook. The message Moses needed to share with the world was valuable, despite his shortcomings. I saw that as a sign. I knew all too well what it felt like to know that I had something to offer yet inadequate in my ability to convey it. Although I was to write my own story, I knew that God has worked through insecurity before, at least since the time of Moses.

As inspired as I felt, it wasn't enough. I still needed another push. I asked God one day, after silently wrestling with my inner desire to write, to give me yet another sign. That night, I received an email. It was from a stranger who had gotten my email from a friend of mine. The mom who emailed me was struggling with transitioning from using pens to a pump. Her daughter was of a similar age to Zandra when she began using a pump, and she was seeking support for this transition. My sign was clear. Although it wasn't strange for me to receive a random email or a call from another mother of a diabetic child, I hadn't had one in a while. The timing was everything. I started to weep with thankfulness for the answered prayer. I knew deep within me that sharing my story would be of value. I realized then how inspired I was by the mothers who had connected with me through the years. They inspired me more than they knew. I began to realize that in order to combat our fears, we needed to come together and share our experiences, just as a photo develops and slowly comes into view. I needed to share my story because I knew that I wasn't the only one who stood by and watched my child navigate life with diabetes. I wanted all other parents who struggle to find their role in their child's disease to know that they are not alone and that their own journey holds precious value.

As people, we are designed to share. Stories have been the way of communication for as long as people have inhabited the world. We learn best through stories, and they serve as a way that shares a message that transcends all barriers. Although I am certainly not the expert on diabetes, I hold the personal story of how it has made an impact in my life.

I am a testament to the knowledge that when we know better, we do better. I know a lot more than I did years ago and I'm a different person, parent, wife and friend because of it. I take comfort that in years to come, I'll look back and see again how much farther I progressed along life's path. I no longer strive for perfection, as I don't require success in the same way that I once did. My worth is already valuable; I don't have to seek it externally or confirm my value with anyone.

When I look back at photos of myself in my younger years, I feel proud. This feeling alone marks one of my greater achievements. I see my old self and hold nothing but compassion for her remarkable effort to do what she thought was best. I see the real love that clung to the belief that more was possible and applaud the hard work that went into the growing pains to metamorphose into something greater.

My old self would feel as though I had to be a part of every moment, feeling guilty when I missed a child's event or even a quiet moment to share. I tried to fill in the blanks of my own discomfort and inadequacies by being very present—perhaps too much so. If I could go back now, I would reach out to the help that was always there and allow those who love me to help shoulder my burden. I would allow those people to walk with me in my fear and be open to their encouragement. If I were to start the journey of diabetes again, I would honour my role as a mother and work on the sidelines to guide and encourage Zandra. I would recognize how fear would erode my confidence and rob me of the joy in my life, all the while deepening my old story of shame. I would allow myself to recognize that I am a part of a greater tapestry whose vibrancy is equally important to the overall picture. I wouldn't allow my failures to define my ability; rather, I would see them as the guidance that they were intended to be.

If I were to start again, I would impart to Zandra the importance of support in our lives. I wouldn't hold her failures as my own; instead, I would show her how to love them, learn from them and let go of them. I would show her how to cry and get angry and love all aspects of herself, including her mistakes. I learned these lessons later than I would have chosen, yet in perfect timing. I now strive to be open and I enjoy the discovery of a new perspective and being receptive to other ideas. I appreciate and have become open to others' experiences without the need to compare or feel regret in my own life. I feel a greater love and peace toward other people than I ever thought possible.

In certain moments I can feel a sense of synchronicity that quietly whispers that I'm exactly where I'm meant to be. This whisper from God doesn't always come in the midst of turmoil, but usually after gaining new perspective after the fact. I listen to these whispers through my intuition—the language of my soul. I have learned to follow these whispers and know that they will lead me to the deeper sense of purpose that I desire in my life.

The value that my own experience has been able to grant me is the assurance that faith is enough. I will never have absolute proof or clarity that assures me I possess all that I need to manoeuvre the minefields in my life and that everything will turn out well. While I want to control everything in my life, I'm aware that only God holds that power. I continue to be tested and I am grateful to know that all I'm here to do is my own part, and I can trust the rest to God. I no longer need to carry the burden of the *ifs* and *hows* in order to move forward. All I need is to trust that I am here for a reason.

Any abuse and pain I have suffered has given me the empathy and other tools I need to identify with others in their own pain and struggles. I sought acknowledgement for the qualities that made me who I am, but was looking for it in all the wrong places. I wanted to be a prodigy, acknowledged for skill, and to have my path set out before me to take the guesswork out of my purpose, but that wasn't to be, as it isn't for most of us. I was called, just as we all are, to fill a role that all the events in our lives have perfectly designed us for, if only we could trust that greater plan.

I want every mother to know that you don't have to feel strong to be strong. You don't have to feel like you're enough to be enough. You are enough just as you are. You need to trust and hold faith that there is a reason for everything and that you are exactly where you are supposed to be. In this exact moment and breath, you can let go and let God guide your next steps. Trust your intuition, as those are His whispers and your way forward. If you miss it, don't worry, God will guide you on your course again.

A diagnosis like diabetes can feel like defeat. It can feel as though the world is conspiring against you and your child. It's easy to question why an innocent child would have to endure the complications day after day.

Diabetes is a disease that separates warriors from the rest. There are no days off from it. At best it is manageable; at worst it's the greatest weight and discouragement that can be felt. A person with diabetes is born with a special purpose. As someone who has walked this path, I see all the mothers, fathers, caregivers and those who struggle with the disease. I understand your pain and desire to give you hope. This bond connects us and serves as a support for those days I lose hope as well. You will never do it alone. My journey has been my gift and moves me toward what I know is my soul's purpose. I have heard my name—I believe.

MEMORIAL
TYLER JORDAN BROZ
(DECEMBER 6, 1998-NOVEMBER 25, 2017)

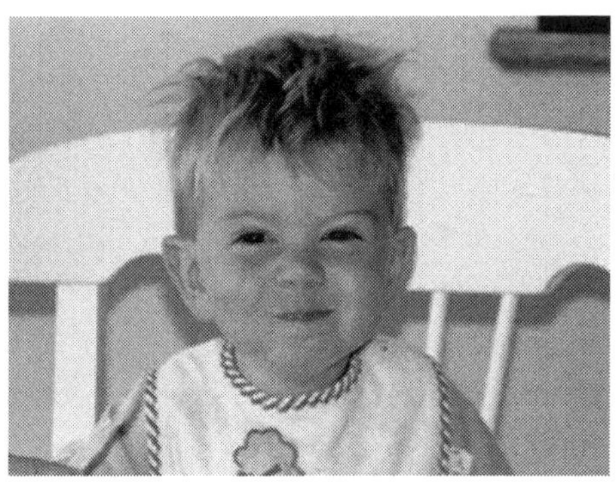

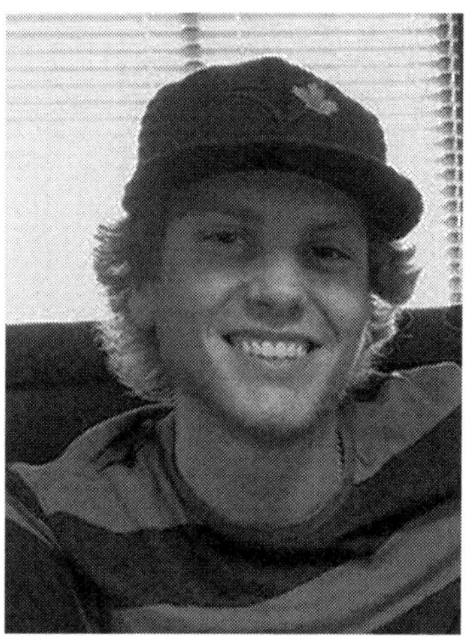

Ty was a people person, just like his dad. Growing up he always had friends over or was at someone's house, begging for sleepovers every weekend, and this didn't change, even after he was diagnosed with diabetes. We made every effort to try to ensure he still did everything he used to do, and to keep life as normal as it had been before it was turned upside down with the diagnosis of a chronic health condition. He continued to play hockey and go to goalie camps; he was a hockey referee at our local arena; he played golf; and he was lucky enough to have travelled to Las Vegas, Washington DC, Thailand, the Philippines, the

Dominican Republic, Costa Rica, Jamaica, the Bahamas and numerous times to Mexico. These holidays are some of our best memories with Ty.

At the time of writing this it has been almost three years since Ty left us. There are two things that stand out when his friends reflect on their times with him: his great smile and his loyal friendship. They recount stories of how Ty was always there when they needed someone to talk to or help them out of a bind. He made sure they got home safely from a party or went to see them when they were feeling sad or lonely—they knew they could always count on him.

His family always remembers his amazing smile, his great sense of humour and his attitude. He loved to spend time with his cousins even though they were older than him, and we all remember fondly the night of playing Cards Against Humanity, when he shocked his mother. For his eighteenth birthday his dad, Ty and I went through his time capsule that we started when he was born, and afterwards he asked if they still made them because he'd like to have one for when he had kids. He will never have a chance to become a husband and a father; we will never know what career path he would have chosen or be able to count on him to look after us in our older years. What we do have are a lot of great memories and the knowledge that he knew how much he was loved.

– Ty's mom and dad, Stephanie and Bruce Broz.

Today we come together,
Our hearts beating as one,
To celebrate the life
Of a soul who died too young.

Talented on the ice, and between the pipes
And always smiling, or sporting a cheeky grin.
There are many memories we'll keep with us
When we think of what could have been.

We'll remember his trips and adventures,
His disease, and the other challenges he faced,
And how regardless of those he lived to the fullest
Ideas of freedom and choices he truly embraced.

We'll miss the fearlessness of his heart,
The purity in his expression of care,
His wonderfully infectious laugh,
And his ridiculous Justin Bieber hair.

He's deeply loved by all of those around him,
The weight of grief feels impossible to bear,
Our forever was such a small moment,
And memories of him are everywhere.

We know he struggled and he fought
With his disease, and through the pain,
What's getting us through this tragedy
Is he'll never have to feel that way again.

We feel the void where he used to be
Yet there's comfort knowing he'll never be truly gone,
Because in all of our hearts he'll always live
And his vibrant and dynamic spirit will carry on.

–Jessica Broz
Ty's cousin who wrote and
read this poem at his funeral.

ACKNOWLEDGEMENTS

Gord: Without your support this book would never have been written. You have guided and loved me throughout every step of Zandra's diabetic journey and kept our family united. You allowed me to share what I needed to express and for me to hold those emotions that were not yet ready to be revealed. Thank you for always seeing my possibility, even when I couldn't see it myself.

Zandra: I believe that before we are born, we choose those whom we share our journey with. Thank you for the honour of being your mom. We have shared many tears, fears and adventures, and I look forward to being there with you for many more. I am so proud to have watched you grow into the divine woman you were born to be.

Olivia: You were born a natural healer and your innate ability to care for others has blessed our family. You stepped in as a natural mother and friend for your siblings and enriched our lives because of your love. This world has a special need for the many gifts you behold.

Joseph: Your easygoing nature has allowed me to always take care of everyone in our home with your full support. You were born with an abundance of understanding and compassion, and a quiet wisdom that has supported our family through many turbulent times. Your love of God and willingness to help anyone in need inspires me every day.

Liam: You haven't known a life without syringe boxes and test strips. Your ever-present joy and humour have helped me to take the most difficult of situations and find lightness within it. You have an ability to know how to raise the spirits of those around you and, in equal measure, offer tenderness when a hug is needed. Inside of me is a book about how each of you inspired and encouraged me to be the best person/mother I could be.

Stollery Children's Hospital: When we first came to the hospital with Zandra, we were immediately met with a genuine love and concern for her and our entire family. Throughout every moment of every year, I knew I could rely upon the help and care of the entire team, to support both physical and emotional needs while we learned how to navigate the ins and outs of diabetes. Words cannot express how blessed we feel to have been able to access the resources and expertise at the Stollery Hospital.

Lion's Foundation of Canada Dog Guides: Thank you for the work that your organization does for so many. It takes special hearts that dedicate themselves to training dogs to enhance the lives of others. I am eternally grateful to everyone at Dog Guides who trained Cinnamon and placed her in our home to work with Zandra. I am ever grateful for the patience and understanding as we worked through the transitions that followed Cinnamon's placement. Cinnamon has been a steadfast companion who, in her ability to love and her desire to work, provided great comfort for our entire family. I marvel at how proud Zandra is to have her vested companion by her side!

Dr. Dhunnoo: Thank you for the genuine care you have shown Zandra. You have always taken a holistic approach to her health that resonated within her spirit. You have shown her how true medicine should be practised. You have inspired her in so many ways, and for that I am eternally grateful.

Laura: Thank you for being my sister. I know that there is nothing you wouldn't do for me and that assurance has supported me throughout my life. You have shown love to our entire family and your guidance has inspired our children to stay close and support one another through life's ups and downs, just as we have done. Thank you for your generosity and kindnesses every day, and your encouragement of me in writing this book. I have always felt at home in your presence.

Karen: Thank you for being my sister. In many ways my story is your story. Your outgoing personality has encouraged me to always look for the fun ways to express myself. You have a creative way of seeing the world around you, and when the three of us sisters get together, we never have a dull moment! Thank you for always encouraging my inner growth and inspiring me to achieve things I never thought possible.

Mary: Thank you for the many dog walks that have been more for us than our pups. It feels only natural that our dogs have become the best of friends and cannot go for long without seeing each other. Your support and advice throughout the years has always helped me to see things from a much lighter and more humorous perspective.

Lina: Thank you for always having my back. Although we live in different countries, distance could never close the gap on us. You have offered me a place to escape to and thoughtful advice that has always been supportive.

Monique: Thank you for your beautiful friendship. No matter how much time goes by between visits, you have always been there when I needed you most. Thank you for sharing your own wisdom with me and always having your kayak ready for a road trip.

Denise: Thank you for setting an example of a warrior woman. The way you have faced your own challenges while being dedicated to your community and keeping a joyful heart has shown me what's possible in my own life.

Cheryl: Thank you for your gift of insight and intuition. There is no question I can ask nor realization I can come to that is beyond your understanding. You have shown me how to be confident with what I know, and how to use it to challenge myself and move forward.

Cinnamon: Although this is something you'll not read, I send you my love and appreciation. You have dedicated your life to loving Zandra as much as I do. Knowing you devote your life to keeping her safe and staying by her side when her heart is heavy has given me untold comfort throughout the years. Thank you from the bottom of my heart.

Mother's everywhere: This book is created out of the universal love that comes from a mother. This love is unique, life-giving and supportive. With this uniqueness, there is a special bond between us that transcends any of our differences. Thank you for everything you do for your children, your families, yourself and the planet. We don't do this mothering alone. We learn from each other and support one another. After all, it takes a village to raise a child.

Manufactured by Amazon.ca
Bolton, ON

15523210R00105